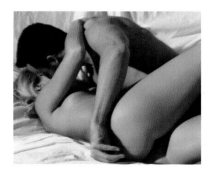

How was it for **YOU**?

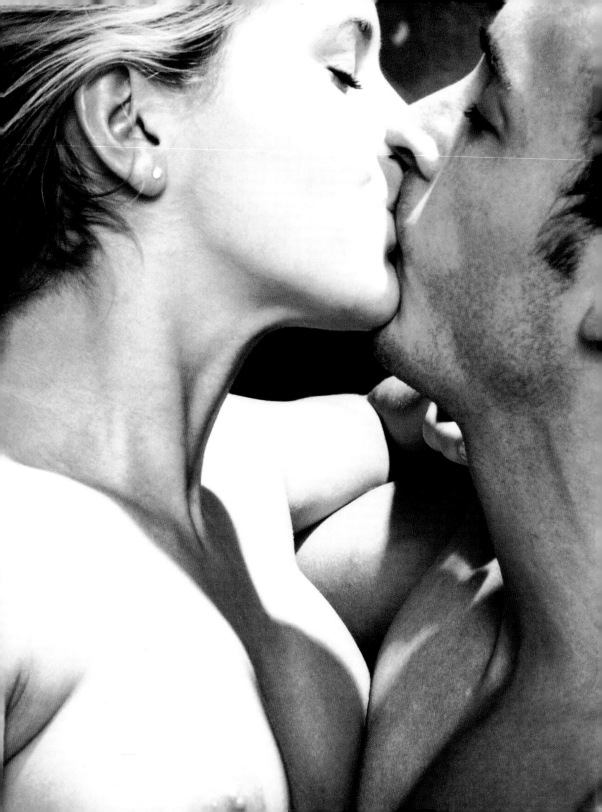

How was it for YOU?

Anne Hooper's guide to making SEX much, much better

Anne Hooper

Carroll & Brown Publishers Limited

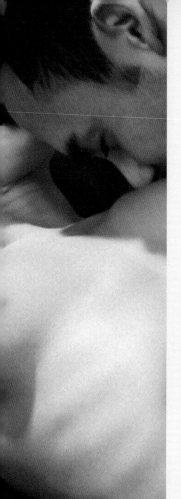

This edition first published in 2005 in the United Kingdom by
Carroll & Brown Publishers Limited
20 Lonsdale Road, London NW6 6RD

Designed by Luis Peral-Aranda

Text copyright © Anne Hooper 2005
Compilation copyright © Carroll and Brown Limited 2005

A CIP catalogue record for this book is available from the British Library.

ISBN 1 904760 07 4

Previous edition published under the title *Sex: The Manual*

10 9 8 7 6 5 4 3 2 1

Reproduced by Colourscan, Singapore
Printed and bound in Spain by Bookprint, S.L., Barcelona

CONTENTS

Introduction

Have you ever asked yourself what is abnormal about fucking in the streets? Or wondered why people who choose not to have sex often get turned into a public joke? Where do our attitudes to sex originally come from? And is it appropriate we should live by them without questioning them? Isn't it just possible that the ideas we accept as 'sexually normal' might actually be harming us?

This manual will start you thinking differently about your sexual attitudes, about the ideas you possess of what is right and wrong. The ideas I am referring to are not the big moral issues, such as those concerning homosexuality or abortion, but the most personal, intimate issues of all – those concerning our deepest being – the gritty dilemma of how we are in bed. How we feel as we wind our legs around another's; whether we dare to look a sex partner in the eye as we fuck; if we feel so free as we twist and writhe that we know we could do literally anything with this lover; these are examples of how we can be. As you look at this list, you may realize that such feelings do not always come automatically. You may reflect that life's grim experience means it is very hard to trust yourself enough to look a partner straight in the eye during sex, let alone trust them.

Human beings have made a fetish out of sex

Somewhere along the line, the idea evolved that sex should be done in private and that anything that intimates public sex, such as public nudity for example, should be made unacceptable. The prohibitions on sex go even further, proscribing how sex should be done, what is good sex and what makes for sexual failure. Instead of just getting on with sex when the mood takes us, we have made a fetish of it. We have trussed it up, garnished, and then refused to eat.

So, what's wrong with fetishes?

Nothing, provided we feel comfortable with them and hurt nobody else with our predilections. But the upshot of our contemporary sexual system is that we feel controlled, indeed we believe we are controlled in bed. If we do not reach orgasm, we believe we are failures. If we find it hard to sustain an erection this becomes a personal reflection on our effectiveness in the world. If we climax too fast we feel out of control. The layer upon layer of fetish wrapping coiled about us makes it ridiculously difficult to take on board a simple fact – that sex is what we make of it. It is perfectly possible to construct sex as a positive or negative experience – any sex. For it is not sex itself which is positive or negative, however wonderful or distressing a particular encounter may be, it is how we choose to feel about it.

Most of us have no idea that there is any choice here. We think that to be miserable in certain circumstances is logical. That is because we are not yet able to see a bigger picture. We cannot, so far, step outside the system of beliefs about sex that we imbibed during our 'civilized' childhood in order to understand that this system of control is only one of many systems. The reality is that we have a choice of systems.

Calming your sex attitudes down

That is where this book comes in. It will start you thinking about your sexual attitudes, specifically about your unconscious ideas on what is right and wrong, so that you can progress to at least contemplating other approaches. By doing so you may be able to see that your present sexual situation has value of its own. You may thus learn to feel better about how things are for you.

But I hope to go further than making you feel better. By bringing a more creative attitude to your sexual relationship, I hope you may discover that you can tackle a number of sexual difficulties, which previously proved intransigent. In this book, each section will work on specific aspects of sex by introducing ideas about how to regard them differently. By reframing your ideas, I hope you see your personal strengths and values emerge from the present-day fog of stress and unhappiness.

I make use of ideas drawn from evolutionary psychology, a school of understanding human behaviour that draws together ideas from cognitive psychology and evolutionary biology. Evolutionary psychology is still developing and many scientists and anthropologists do not agree with its ideas, most notably Hilary and Steven Rose as expounded in their book *Alas Poor Darwin*. The Roses may be proved right but that doesn't mean that it isn't healthy to rethink your position on sex – pun definitely intended. This book is all about rethinking your position.

Anne J Hooper

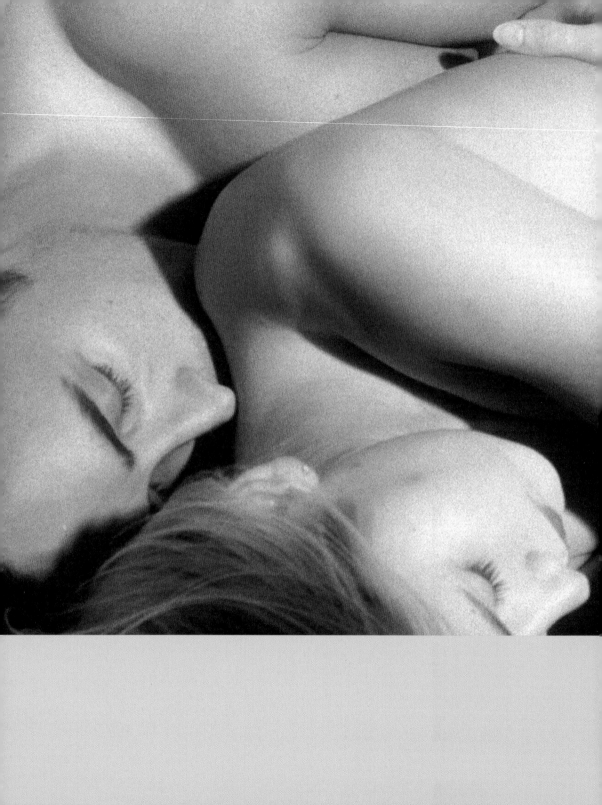

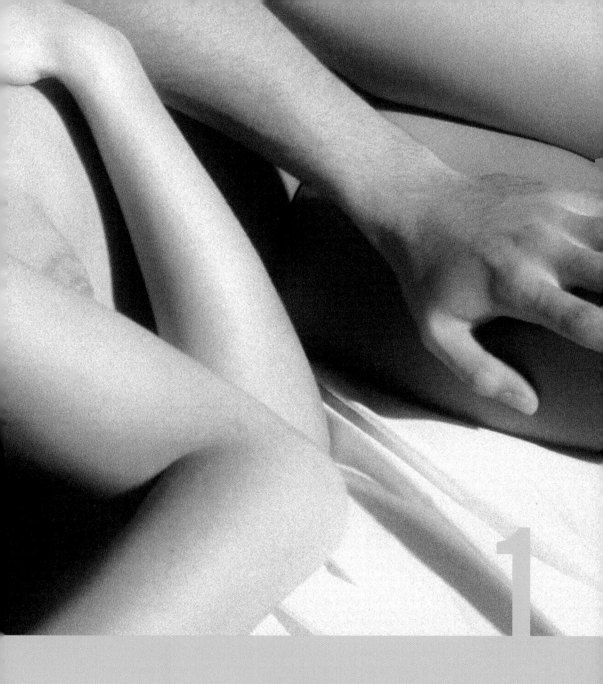

1

Growing Our Beliefs

Where Do Ideas About Sex Come From?

The famous Viennese inventor of Adlerian psychology, Alfred Adler, believed that personality is shaped first by our experience within the immediate family, later by the wider context of larger family and friends and ultimately by the bigger outside world. Today we might add a fourth dimension to the growth of personality by including global influences (i.e. the impact of worldwide telecommunications that brings ideas and customs of just about every nation to our door).

Adler believed that humans are subject to a basic drive towards gaining a sense of personal value, since our earliest experiences (as babies) are of feeling small and weak in a world of giants. Out of this desire to feel strong comes the need to believe we are effective in this world and that other people see us and respect us as such. It is through this process that we begin to grow a belief system.

Sex and Parents

So where does sex fit into this? We learn not just about the facts of life (and sex) from parents but we also see the example of warmth, trust and communication that they set. If we have parents who fight like mad, but who then make up, retire to the bedroom and come out the next day looking happy, we learn that good sex is vitally re-affirming. Ergo – sex is strengthening.

If our parents are able to be open about sex, to discuss it honestly with us when we are infants, by the time we grow up we feel reasonably comfortable with sex when we finally get to it. Interestingly, research shows that the more open a parent is able to be with children about sex, the older they are likely to be before having first-time sex, the more likely to use contraception and the less likely to conceive uninvited babes. The logic here is that knowing about sex allows us to feel secure and confident.

If sex is never discussed, and/or there is a sense of tension and strain between parents, young men and women grow up to believe that sex can be full of problems. This doesn't appear to put them off having sex but it does mean that they know less about it, less about their own sexual response and are much less confident as individuals.

An example of this latter situation was seen in the young women who used to take part in my sexuality workshops in the 1970s and 1980s. Many of them found it difficult to experience orgasm partly due to a serious lack of personal self-esteem. These women

In the absence of information, and where there is a tense atmosphere concerning sex, we are forced to make up the facts for ourselves and what we imagine is more stressful than what we really know.

regularly described fathers who were cold and distant, and mothers who were timid, nervous and who found it impossible to stand up to their partner's bad temper and moods (i.e. stressful parental example and little sexual information).

Social and Sexual Teaching

Hand-in-hand with parental influence goes positive social and sexual teaching. In the 1970s and 1980s very few women in my groups had ever been told about:

- Taking time over beginning a sexual friendship;
- Taking time over mutually discovering sex;
- How orgasm actually worked;
- Possessing a clitoris.

Today's young men and women know rather more about sexual behaviour than those of 25 years ago thanks to the burgeoning of sexual advice in the media and also thanks to the partial breakdown of inhibition over discussion between parents and children. Yet many of today's budding sexual beings still don't appear to know that for sex to work well it helps to establish a caring, loving friendship.

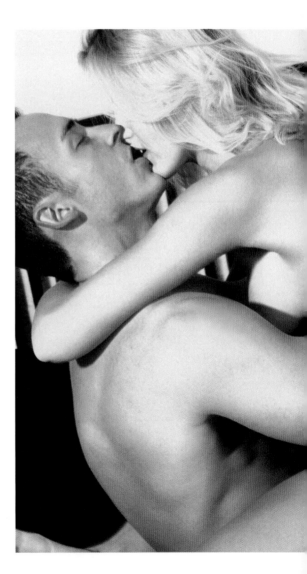

It seems that most youngsters can talk to their peers but few do so with their parents and learning about anything from your peers has its pluses and minuses. The pluses are that you are likely to give and receive information on a level you can truly relate to and understand; the minuses are that the information itself may be faulty or biased in directions that prove uncomfortable or even emotionally harmful.

So it's possible to learn how to do sex from receiving sexual ideas from people of your own age group but not to know how to enjoy it.

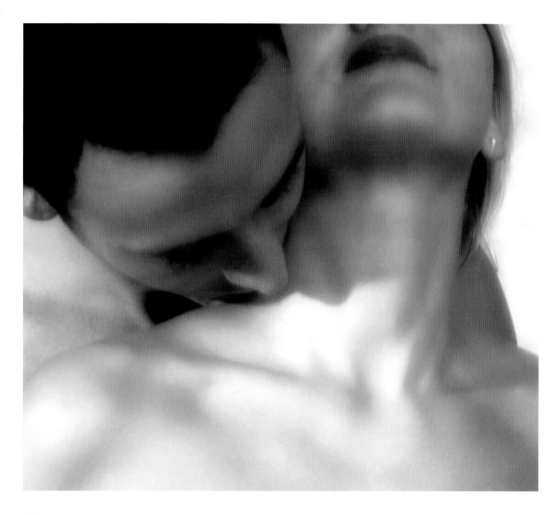

Origins of Sexual Ideas

And what about those ideas? What about the concepts we take on board from parents, school or peers? Where do those ideas actually hail from originally? I don't mean which textbook did they arise from. Nor do I mean which parent or teacher expounded them. I mean where did the ideas actually originate?

The Common Sense View

The answer is a simple one, say the socio-biologists. Sex is a human instinct. Genitals are equipped with amazing sensations that virtually compel individuals to explore and to use their superior primate intelligence to subsequently fit an erect penis into a vagina. Sex is also an animal instinct and primitive cave people, living alongside other species, were perfectly capable of seeing these other creatures mate and of transferring such visual information to their own species and following suit. The present-day experience of sex must, therefore. have had its origins in this early time and developed accordingly.

Since, in evolutionary terms, there appeared no need for female orgasms, it was widely believed for years that women didn't have them. As recently as 1975, certain English doctors denied the possibility of female orgasm on the grounds that since women didn't ejaculate, orgasm was therefore impossible. Now that it has been proved beyond doubt that women do experience the big 'O', biologists and anthropologists have been dreaming up evolutionary reasons why.

One explanation is that at the moment of orgasm, the cervix (i.e. the entrance to the uterus) dips and bathes in the pool of ejaculated semen lying there inside the vagina, thus expediting the journey of sperm towards ovum. Ergo, women were equipped with orgasm in order to perpetuate the species. I would hazard a guess and go further. Since a primitive cave woman may well have been subjected to the rapacious sexual advances of many males, it may be that the experience of orgasm favoured the sperm of the men who most turned her on. Her babies would be those of the men with whom she could develop the richest sexual relationships.

We have absolutely no idea about intimate relationships between such early men and women. However, all the new research into genetic identity and the brain seems to tell us that these ancient lovers were probably not that different from you and me. They didn't have much technology, they had an appalling struggle to survive in the wild but their brains were probably not all that different.

The Evolutionary View

Charles Darwin, author of *The Descent of Man* and *Selection in Relation to Sex* is probably the most influential determinator of sexual thinking in the past and present centuries. He had at least two major theories about evolution. The first was the idea of natural selection and the second was the idea of sexual selection.

PRIMITIVE SEX

Scientists are of the opinion that primitive man was naturally a premature ejaculator since it would have aided his survival in a cruel world to get sex over and done with fast. If you know that a sabre tooth tiger just might be hanging around the entrance to your cave, it's not a good idea to have your back turned for too long. So today's premature ejaculators, far from feeling ashamed of their sexual prowess, might feel proud that they are true men in an absolutely fundamental sense.

Cave men who became impotent may well have been those who were stressed, diseased, ageing or just plain worn out. It might have suited them to be forced to take a break from sex regardless of their opinion in the matter; it might have suited their equally ageing partners; and it might have suited the quality of the resultant sperm, ensuring that below-par sperm did not result in below-par babies – we're talking gene transfer here.

The compulsive genes The theory of natural selection has it that human brains and therefore human beings evolved through survival of the fittest. In other words, if you could survive well enough and long enough to father or mother as many children as possible, those children were most likely to be survivors in their own right and to continue to pass on your genes. Your line would thus survive, thanks to its constant and ultimate fitness at adapting and coping with the hideously difficult circumstances into which you were born.

The men and women who coped less well were likely to be snuffed out by a falling tree, eaten by a predator or, most important of all, kicked down to a lower position in society and therefore given less access to mates. On these bases there are probably not a lot of descendants of the less able alive and well in the world today.

The problem with the theory of natural selection left on its own is that it doesn't explain the very important differences between man and the other great primates. Chimpanzees, gorillas and other great apes also have survived and share 98 per cent of their DNA with us, their cousins. Yet they didn't make the great leap whereby their brains enlarged and they developed the major and detailed skill of speech. (They may be in the process of doing that now but only with help from us. They haven't done it on their own.)

What is more, alongside speech developed the creative arts. From a purely biological point of view, the great arts seemed to be useless – a kind of sideline that is a dead end from the point of view of survival. One biological argument went that because our enlarged brains gained the ability to learn new things, all these extras were merely 'frosting on the cake'. Yet today new ideas about sexuality and creativity are suddenly hitting the headlines. I quote here Geoffrey Miller who in his book *The Mating Mind* makes a compelling argument for the additional evolution of the second type of selection coined by Darwin – 'sexual selection'.

Sexual selection It is not quite what you might imagine. It doesn't simply mean that men and women choose the partner who most turns them on and so passes the most sexually successful genes on down through that particular line. Of course, it does mean that, but it means a lot more beside. It offers an explanation of why human beings write, paint, think, tell stories, do anything that might interest and intrigue others. It may be connected to the sexual hoops we put ourselves through in the here-and-now. It certainly offers explanations for our choices to confine ourselves to one mate instead of many, or at least make a show of doing so. It might underlie the fact that we often believe we ought to do sex in a certain way, in a certain room, with or without clothes, in a 'good' or a 'bad' fashion. And since these beliefs may be responsible for undermining our instincts about sex, it's worth taking a look at their origins.

Sexual selection through mate choice is an important theory because, argues Miller, it doesn't only explain peacocks, or indeed any other kind of decoration or embellishment, be it appearance, humour or story-telling, it also explains how and why the brain enlarged so massively, marking us out so definitively from other species.

'Before language evolved, our ancestors could not easily perceive one another's thoughts, but once language had arrived, thought itself became the subject of sexual selection.' (Miller) Sexual selection may actually have been responsible for the development of language. Miller describes a positive self-feedback loop, driven by that most powerful of sensual urges. To put it simply, sexual preference reinforces developing language which, in turn, reinforces sexual preference.

If a human primate female constantly selects the male whose grunts and growls are most interesting to her, over the centuries those grunts and growls transform into language.

WHY THE PEACOCK SPREADS HIS TAIL

Geoffrey Miller explains his point through a description of a peacock and why it evolved its gorgeous tail. Such a huge appendage might well be seen, from a survival of the fittest point of view, as an evolutionary disadvantage since it must mean that a peacock would find it exceedingly difficult to flee from a predator. Since peacocks remain with us today, there must be some other advantage to be derived from such over-the-top, exotic personal decoration. Miller's theory is that the beautiful tail developed over the eons because peahens liked them; because peahens favoured male peacocks with a wonderful display over dull, ordinary males with little or no display. This is what Darwin described as sexual selection through mate choice.

What is more, the male who displays the most versatile courtship is also likely to display the most health, intelligence and fitness – all evolutionary advantages. Humour, rated highly in today's psychological tests of desirable partner traits, would have evolved simultaneously since humour would give an edge to ordinary speech. The humorous partner would gain an advantage over the less amusing partner.

Miller's theory is strenuously opposed by some scientists, most notably Steven and Hilary Rose. Their view is that the theory is too general and that there are too many assumptions to make it meaningful. Yet Miller makes an interesting point when he states that, for thousands of years, early hominids continued perfectly well without evolving this highly sophisticated brain. Brain size only tripled in our ancestors between two and a half million and a hundred thousand years ago. If it were only natural selection that was driving us, he believes, we wouldn't have needed anything extra.

Natural selection accounts for our survival as hominids. But it needs something else to explain that sudden leap in brain size. Miller argues that sexual selection does this. He writes 'Sexual selection through mate choice is a fickle, unpredictable, diversifying process. It takes species that make their livings in nearly identical ways and gives them radically different sexual ornaments. It never happens the same way twice. It drives divergent rather than convergent evolution.' By this theory, it is sexual selection that enlarges the brain in the first place and then accounts for the subsequent development of creativity and imagination, for it was only in the last one hundred thousand years that men began to grow civilized.

Another reason why the theory of sexual diversity through mate selection may have found it hard to be taken seriously is because it depends on conceding to women the power to shape men – not the other way round. Or at least it does when applied to animals. With humans it seems highly likely that sexual selection is a two-way process.

So how does sexual selection theory affect the experience of penis in vagina today? Surely, evolved or otherwise, actual heterosexual intercourse always did consist of penis in vagina, give or take a few variations? We come back to a point made at the beginning of this section on sexual selection. Perhaps today's constraints about sex, all those 'beliefs' that there are right ways and wrong ways of doing it, all those orgasmic hurdles men and women feel forced to jump through, perhaps all of these are forms of evolutionary test. If you apply the sexual selection theory to our most intimate life, we could be weeding out the partners who are unsuited to the evolution of our line.

Of course, in this day and age, there aren't many guarantees that a partner who does inspire trust and with whom you have a good open sex life, will be a good long-term parent either. But at least his or her attractions get the chance to be passed on through his or her share of your child's genetic make-up.

If you feel uncomfortable and uneasy with one partner in bed, the odds are there will be some discomfort and unease in other parts of the relationship. Would this be the person you want as parent to your children? Answer: probably not.

Civilizing influences So restraints on sex, even sex problems, might be evolutionary tests. If you get the answer to them right (i.e. if you manage to sort out the sex problem and overcome the communication difficulties), you pass the test. If you fail, that's it. Your joint line is doomed. It could be a powerful method of weeding out the wrong partners.

Sex is an immensely powerful drive. One of the fears that today's humans have about dropping some of their inhibitions or prohibitions about sex is that, in the lack of these restraining modern influences, 'they might go mad and turn into wild animals'. Since by evolution's standards we are only in a second stage of evolutionary development, there may be some real truth lying behind such a fear. Who is to say that, let off the leash, we won't become our instinctive ancestors, rather than our thinking contemporary selves? We certainly seem to see this where aggression is concerned. Behaviour in a crowd for example, often overrides normal inhibition so that we act seemingly out of character. A football match or a pop concert is an excellent example. Yet not all such 'primitive' behaviour is 'bad'. Exuberance, enthusiasm, sexual expression, might be termed 'good'. The fact that these are expressed in ways not generally termed 'civilized' does not necessarily down rate such qualities.

Most sex therapists would prefer to see a little more of the overriding exuberance of the cave when it comes to sex and a lot less of the restraining influences of so called civilisation. Where primitive man might not have given a thought to his partner's orgasm, he may have possessed enough staying power and intelligence to want to prolong the good sensations of love-making. With this as a possible desire he may have kept going long enough and strong enough for his partner to climax. Naturally this is pure speculation. We can have absolutely no idea of how sex was for our ancient ancestors.

What is certain is that if sexual selection by mate choice, is responsible for the kind of sex we get today, we humans have not yet selected mates for their ability to provoke exquisite and infallible sexual enjoyment!

This is a way of saying that our present enjoyment of what goes on in bed is stuck somewhere between the old and the new. Instead of just getting on with what intercourse offers, we make a song and dance about it. Instead of moving on to a more satisfactory sexual mate, we often feel stuck with the present one. Instead of accepting that some men and women prefer multiple matings, we tell ourselves fiercely that possession of the other person is all.

Jealousy, a powerful instinctive feeling, tells us to hang on fiercely to what (or who) we consider our territory yet, at the same time, natural sexual desire tells us how nice it would be to make love to Brad Pitt, Beyoncé Knowles, Jennifer Aniston or George Clooney. Instead of tearing each other's clothes off in the street and coupling at the time we most feel like it, we bottle up those feelings and take them home where only hours later we can do something with them, and then discover that, what bad luck, the moment has passed.

It's worth bearing in mind that we are still in the process of evolution. We will always be in the process of evolution; hence the uncertainties, the need to feel secure when in actuality we can never be completely secure. These are some of the conflicts between our primitive side and our sophisticated one. And to make life even more interesting, I should explain that 'sexual selection' is not the only theory that affects how we think about sex.

There is another newer theory that allows us to see things from another viewpoint.

Memes

One rare ability that humans share with only a very few other creatures is the ability to imitate. Apes, dolphins, certain whales, a few birds and rats can do this, too, and because they can, we rate them amongst the most highly intelligent species on this planet, second only to us.

When you imitate, something has been passed on. It may be an idea, a story, a type of behaviour, the way you move your arms when you are enthusiastic, no matter what.... Whatever it is that has been imitated has now been given a name. This 'something' has been named a 'meme'. Richard Dawkins, author of *The Selfish Gene*, first mentioned it in 1976 but psychologist Susan Blackmore got to thinking about the idea of memes during a long recuperation from illness and the result was her fascinating book *The Meme Machine*.

Her chapters on memes and sex are particularly pertinent. She begins by making a point that sex, power and food are evolutionary powerful subjects and that one of the reasons we see so many books about sex (and food) is that we are still driven by these primitive drives. Our present-day brains have evolved to focus specifically on such vital interests. In addition, stories, items of information, films, photographs – anything that presses the sex button – are also memes, for what are these all but methods of repeating, informing and replicating information.

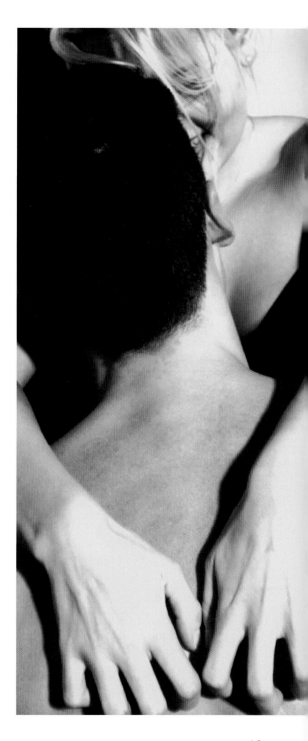

A kind of 'ideas virus' But Blackmore goes much further when she theorises that all modern sexual behaviour is meme-driven. Many memes are passed from parent to child, such as how to eat cleanly and how to pass the butter. Children also get their first language from their parents and, in so doing, rely entirely on the power of imitation. What we have to get our head round here is that it is not only the information which is passed on, but also the meme. Blackmore sees a meme as a kind of 'ideas virus' with a mission to survive, just as genetic material has a mission to survive. A successful meme is an idea, which has survived in some form or other, since the beginning of intelligent hominids.

But... and it's a big but... like any other information it changes as it gets passed from one person to another. We've all played the game of Chinese Whispers, where the whispered information that arrives at the far end of the line is often very different from the information that first started off.

There are three main methods of transferring memes, says Blackmore. One is 'vertical transmission', where information is passed on neatly from parent to child. Then there is 'horizontal transmission', which is between peers, for example, the sort of sex information

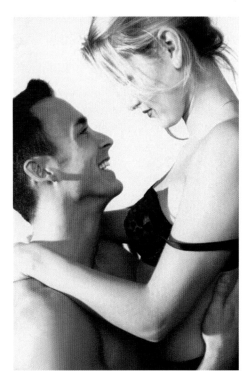

that we talked about earlier. Third is 'oblique transmission', such as that between an uncle and a nephew or between an older and a younger cousin.

The 'vertical' sex meme The reason the type of transmission matters is because in this first meme, the ideas get handed on alongside the genetic material. In other words, we will continue to learn and adapt just as our family always has for generation after generation. If we apply this to sex, we might, for example, continue to believe that sex should only be confined to the partner we marry; that we shouldn't experience sex before the wedding; that sex should be done in the privacy of the marriage bed, probably at the weekends when we are not tired out; that sex is merely one of many aspects of family life. Because this is a lifestyle that has suited the family up till now, there will be little conflict involved for the individual in doing sex this way.

The 'horizontal' sex meme When memes are transmitted horizontally (i.e. between school friends or work colleagues), there is no guarantee that the ideas themselves will match the family ideas, so new notions are brought in which, although they may be exciting, will also be in conflict both with family values and perhaps even with our own inner sense of what is safe and what isn't.

A crude sexual example would be the young man from a traditional family who is invited to a group sex party. He may want to take part and may get turned on by the excitement, but he may also feel out of his depth and be forced to get very drunk in order to cope. His new memes are in conflict with his old. And what will now be transmitted to the next generation – the new or the old? So the ideas themselves become embattled. Which meme will win?

Susan Blackmore feels that in modern society, where memes can be transmitted very rapidly by the media or the internet, our way of life is transforming very fast indeed. The success of an idea today depends on its speedy transmission. In future, therefore it will be the rapidly versatile who will do best rather than the steady, sure plodders.

The 'oblique' sex meme Similar to the 'vertical', in that transmission is between family members, though lying further away, there is, however, a greater potential for new notions being applied to sex, though this is most likely between individuals of a similar age group like cousins. And, as families become more widespread, it is possible that famly concepts of sex will broaden.

Memes and marriage Many of the memes, which we are in the process of discarding, are to do with ensuring the survival of the family line – keeping the family gene pool pure. The idea of marriage, the horrible punishments for adultery, the notion that monogamy is better than other marriage practises contribute to these. This latter is particularly interesting because it appears to be inaccurate.

What I think Susan Blackmore is speculating about, although she doesn't actually state it, is the possibility that the spreading of one's own ideas, to a point where you might even influence the world view, may be a basic instinctive drive in itself. Some people are independently taking such notions very seriously indeed. The Gorbachev World Peace Forum, formed some eight years ago, meets every September to formulate ideas, which it hopes to transmit into the ether as an attempt to promote world peace. On the basis of the meme theory, there is sound reason behind such a plan.

Memes and intimacy So what are the connections between memes and the intimacy of sex? The intimacy of sex is such that it lends itself to the sharing of ideas. Beautiful female Mata Haris have traditionally used the bed as a method of extracting secret information. But perhaps more relevant to readers of this book is the connection between stories, ideas and scenarios acted out as a prelude to the sex act. This type of sexual prelude may have come to us from peers rather than parents. We may not yet feel entirely comfortable with it, but almost certainly, sex games are here to stay.

> *Many of us are highly resistant to the idea of new*
> *sex practises, feeling swamped or out of our depth.*
> *This doesn't mean that we are not interested.*

Sex is a powerful trigger – most of us would love to learn more. One method of dealing with a meme too far would consist of inventing a meme of our own. If sex systems are up for grabs, if truly anything goes, the world would be able to cope with what we can come up with, too. Of course, there will always be doubters and condemners. And we can feel confident about our own ideas instead of ashamed. Ex-President Clinton, in the face of enormous disapproval has managed it. Yet not everyone has thought this through. We need to take on board enough self-confidence to believe such a self-based thought. It is not other people who are the problem. We are the problem.

Very few of us actually see other people doing sex. It isn't customary in the West to view parents coupling. This means that we have no practical example to follow. From a meme point of view this means that our meme of doing sex is incomplete. When we actually get down to fucking, we operate from having heard or read about the act, perhaps having seen pictures, occasionally films, but never, of course, knowing anything about the feelings involved.

We bring to early sexual experience therefore a combination of incomplete ideas plus instinct. How we actually relate to A.N. Other therefore, how intimate we manage to become, is one of the few things we make up for ourselves.

We literally invent sexual experience, albeit one based on theories fed into us by parents and culture. Some of us manage it with artistry, some with enough ease for

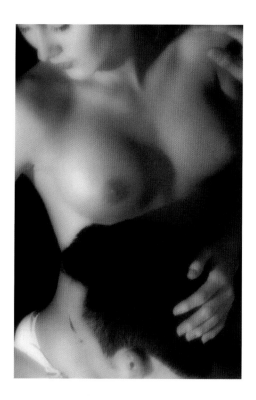

pleasurable enjoyment, and some of us make a complete balls-up. I come back therefore to the thought that since we actually invent part of our sexual experience, we can re-invent it, too. Or we can build on the invention, extending its parameters. It is OUR experience, not someone else's. And if we want to change it therefore, we can.

POLYANDRY IS GOOD FOR YOU!

Blackmore writes of a group of people living in the high Himalayas who practise fraternal polyandry. One woman marries two or more brothers who inherit the family land. Studies of this group have shown that their system does, in fact, maximize their genetic fitness. Grandmothers with polyandrous daughters were found to have more surviving offspring that those with monogamous daughters This system is founded upon the idea handed down from generation to generation (vertical) that survival is maximized by such an arrangement. Sadly however, the arrangement is now breaking down. As such remote villages come into contact with the rest of civilization, ideas of work and marriage change. Such is the power of horizontal transmission.

New Brain Research

Another avenue that offers up-to-date ideas about how to handle life is current research and thinking about the brain. Through further understanding of how the human brain works, we are getting a new handle on how to think about sex. Neuroscientists believe that the left brain contains an area, which has been dubbed the 'interpreter'. The right brain is a type of automatic brain, which lets us respond to stimuli in what feels like an instinctive manner. The instincts may have come from the evolutionary years prior to consciousness when we reacted automatically to certain stimuli.

An example of how the right brain responds to sexual stimuli is this: when a male sees a pretty woman with long legs and a short skirt walk past, he usually cannot help his instinctive reaction of arousal or, at the very least, appreciation.

Getting Stuck in the Missionary Position

The interpreter in our left brain allows us to build on strong bursts of neuronal activity, such as pleasure or pain, increasing the build-up to become a belief that, for example, the missionary position is one of the most pleasurable ways of experiencing sex.

Factors that will have been taken in and unconsciously weighed by the interpreter in the left brain will be: the intimacy of full frontal sexuality; the easy access to each other's pleasure zones, especially to the clitoris; the proximity of the sensually laden lips to those of your mate. In the early months of a relationship, the missionary position will get honed to perfection so that it delivers the goods in the most satisfactory manner possible.

Next, the missionary sex routine crosses over from the left brain, where it has been constructed and 'interpreted', to the right brain where your way of having sex is now stored as a 'given'. From now on, the way you do sex will be virtually automatic. You will unconsciously go, most often, to doing sex in the missionary position. It has become instinctive. It has been established in your right brain pathways as your sex pattern. (For further details about this, see Susan Greenfield's *The Human Brain – A Guided Tour*.)

On reading this, you may feel indignant. 'Of course I have sex in a variety of patterns,' you think with irritation. 'There is no one way in which I experience sex. I am a thinking, conscious human being with choices in this life.'

Brain science would have us think that all choices are limited by the premise that any thoughts and beliefs we hold are founded upon the very first primitive firing of neurones.

We're talking about those sparks of brain activity our millions of times great-grandparents experienced when they coupled with the entire tribe or even when they masturbated as they sat high up in a tree. Most people hate this analogy, rejecting it fiercely. But if you try the experiment of allowing yourself to contemplate it, it can be helpful.

Deep down there is an animal inside us, albeit an extremely bright one. Why should it hurt to get in touch with that animal? The civilized newer layer of the brain is not going to allow you to run amok.

How Sex in the Brain Works

It might feel safer to get in touch with the 'animal inside' if you knew a little more about the way in which the sex centres of the brain work. An incredibly simplified description would be to say that the little grey cells transmit chemical messengers called hormones to other cells. Each hormone transmits a different message. If you see someone who turns you on, your brain sends out chemicals that get you into sexual mode, so that you lubricate and get a mini erection of the clitoris if you are female, or gain a penile erection if you are male.

But, unfortunately for our understanding of it, the brain then gets much trickier. Sex researchers at the Kinsey Institute are beginning

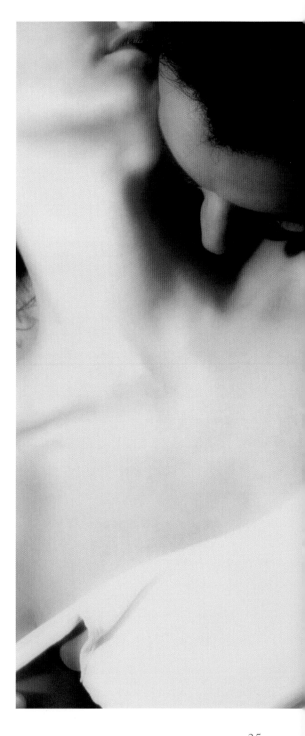

OVER-CONTROLLING INHIBITION

Other problems where this in-balance might be the cause, are the widower who can't make love to his new partner because he feels he is being unfaithful to his late wife. His emotions cause his inhibition. Then there is the mother who can't relax in bed because she fears her toddler will wander into the bedroom. She clearly has a concrete reason for feeling inhibited.

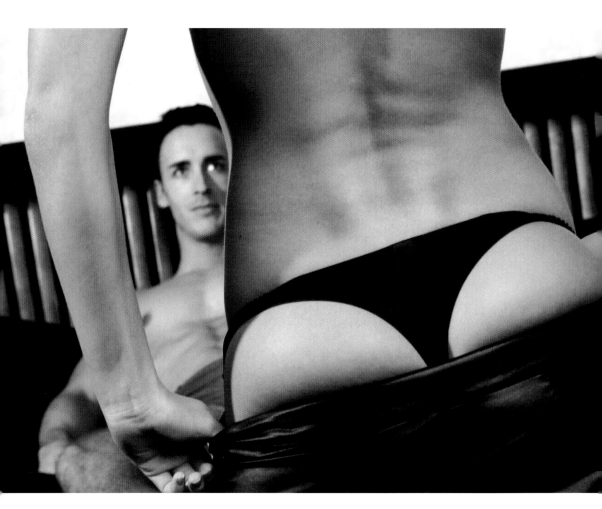

to believe that the brain contains at least two centres, possibly three, that balance sex feelings. The first centre is an 'excitor', an area that pretty obviously gives rise to sexual excitement (i.e. arousal). The second centre is an 'inhibitor', an area that clamps down on feelings of sexual excitement and prevents arousal. The two work in combination to provide a balanced sexual behaviour. The inhibitor preventing you from becoming overtly sexy in inappropriate surroundings. The third is also an 'inhibitor' although scientists are not yet so sure about this one. They reckon it might explain why some people experience a kind of global shutdown of sexual feelings.

Balancing excitement and inhibition However, the ratio of excitement to inhibition can go wrong. Ex-President Clinton is an example of a man who suffered from too much excitement and not enough inhibition. This means that, from time to time, he behaved sexually in a way that is considered to be unacceptable to American society. It is highly likely that it is his sexual brain centres that were directing this behaviour rather than his conscious choice.

Some of the women in my sexuality therapy groups found it so difficult to turn on that they couldn't climax with their partner even though they wanted to. These women probably suffered from an overactive dose of inhibition. But we proved in the group that if you work on overcoming the inhibition, sexual desire really does get a chance to gleam through. In the 1970s and 1980s, we used therapeutic methods that involved gaining trust, reading sexually stimulating material, even watching sexy films. Today, there are pills that work much faster and that regulate these two centres. Viagra helps men get erections although it may not give them desire while Phentolamine can lower inhibition. Neither drug, however, is suitable for everyone though. Beta-blockers lower anxiety levels and slow sexual response. Moreover, sex therapy can work at raising levels of sexual excitement and lower anxiety so that inhibition doesn't cut in so fast as it did with the women in my sexuality groups.

General mood also affects sexual response. Anxiety, fear, anger and depression play their part but since the next section focuses on how preconceived ideas affect our sexual receptivity, mood will be fully described there.

Appraisal

We are in the middle of a major upheaval in our sexual thinking. If the theory of memes is correct, memes have spread to a point where they are truly breaking down established patterns while other sex patterns are being bandied about. This can be both exciting and scary. How can we know how to judge anything? What will constitute a good sexual relationship? Does any of this matter anyway? After all, however you choose to think about it, heterosexual sex continues to consist of putting penis into vagina, doesn't it?

Improving Mental Attitudes

The Moon Story, described opposite, is a parable for our times. And is, of course, intended as a joke. Yet there is a chunk of the story that remains important. We are the only people who can have our experience; no one else can do it for us. We encounter external events specific to us, which affect how we ultimately live our life because such experiences alter our brain make-up. If we have been molested or raped as a young teenager, we are not going to feel the same about subsequent sex as the young man or woman who chooses the exact time and circumstances in which to enjoy safe, pleasurable sensuality for their first time. Mental attitudes to sex are changed by external events. Yet mental attitudes can be improved.

Change does not only have to come from the external or from the unpleasant. We can change through gaining knowledge. We can change by deliberately putting ourselves in the path of certain memes. We can change thanks to extreme pleasure – a fact not often noted by psychotherapists although this constitutes the main working premise for sex therapists. We can change by taking seriously old ideas from former times instead of discarding them on the grounds that old means out of date. We can change by taking on new ideas that offer us new perspectives. We can change by daring to open ourselves up to experience that would not be a traditional choice. Who is to say, for example, that the swingers of the 1970s experienced poor-quality sexuality?

Many people would say certainly not, but they cannot know. They cannot be in the brains of those people. When swingers say that they gain a powerfully effective eroticism, a vital sense of freedom, an actual orgasmic experience that is multiplied in strength, they could be absolutely right. No one else can experience their feelings so no one else can know if they have discovered some kind of sensuality that has escaped the rest of us.

All very well, you might argue, but swingers possess the temperament that allows them to cope with swinging. If you don't have the temperament, you won't have positive experiences.

True again, but temperament isn't everything. Opening up to experiment is part of the picture. Please understand, I am not making a compelling argument for the whole world to start swinging. (I'd go to the barricades to protest against any enforced sexual beliefs.) But I am attempting to explain that a different mindset leads to different experiences – even if ultimately they are based on continuing to revolve around the earth.

Which leads me on to the next section of the book. In order to open yourself up to anything different, new or potentially threatening, it is necessary to rid yourself of preconceived fears and prejudices. Chapter Two offers some thoughtful exercises on just how to do that.

THE MOON GOES IN FOR THERAPY

Did you hear the story about the Moon going around the Earth?

The Moon discovered psychotherapy. It went in for long and intensive counselling sessions. When it finally emerged, it did, it explained, feel quite different. Whereas previously it had revolved thoughtlessly around and around the Earth, now, the Moon disclosed proudly, it chose to do so.

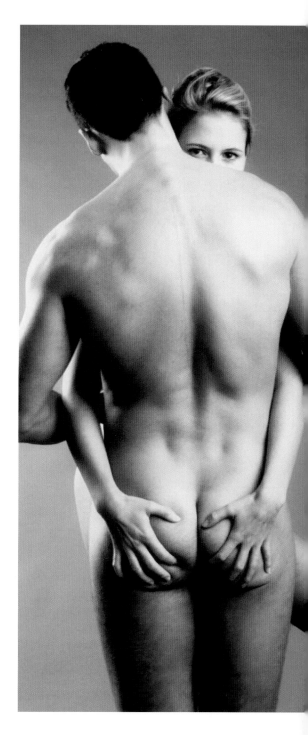

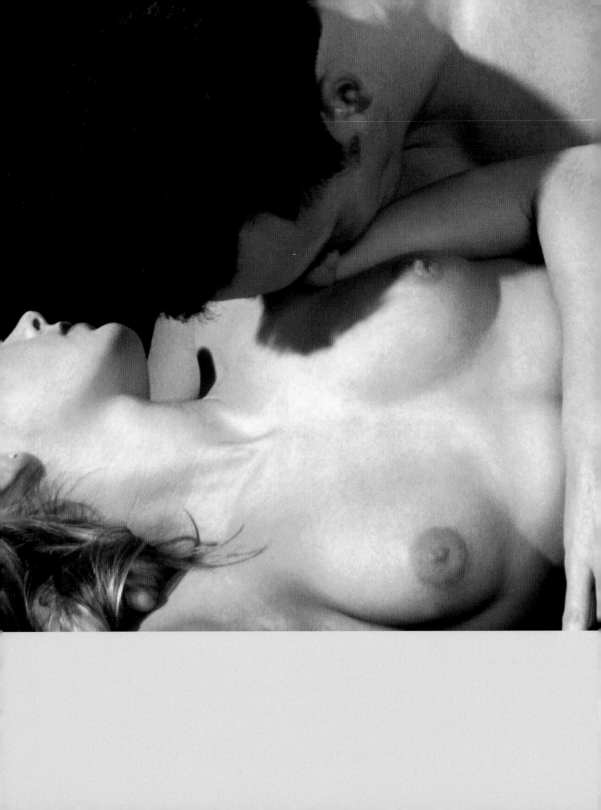

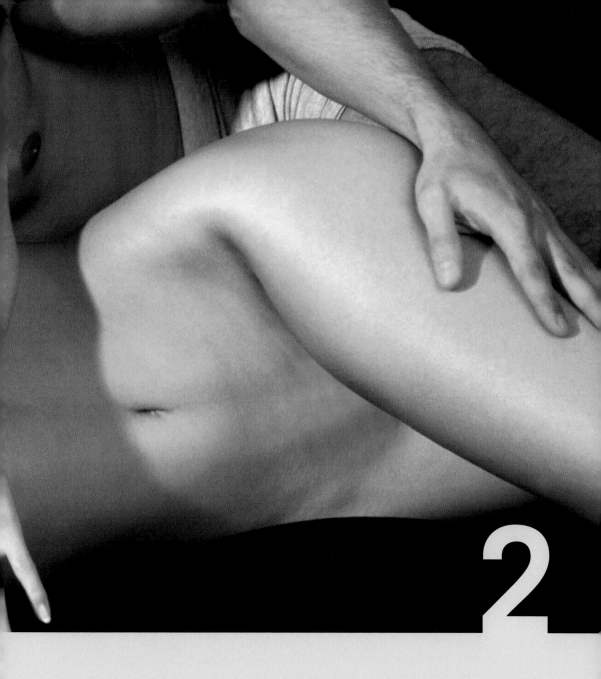

2

Moods and Emotions

Strong Feelings

Moods and emotions play a big part in the experience of sex. This sounds so obvious that you probably wonder why I even bother stating it. The reason lies in new information about the brain. There is now a strong suspicion that areas of the brain, which deal with strong emotion, may be situated next to areas that deal with sex. It seems highly likely that one 'little grey cell' can literally seep its intelligence into and over to the next ones.

So this means that if, for example, you are deeply depressed, your sex centres get depressed, too, thus making it difficult to get turned on. If you are prone to deep-seated anxiety, your sex drive may get anxious too and need to be reassured over and over again by the sex act itself. Most people might probably think that if an individual is anxious, the sex act itself would become fraught with anxiety and suffer. But surprisingly sexological studies have proved virtually the opposite.

Anxiety

Professor John Bancroft, author of *Human Sexuality and its Problems*, studied men who were told they would be given an electric shock if they produced an erection. You might expect such unfortunates to become extremely anxious and to respond by wilting in all directions. But no! Eight out of the 10 men studied showed that it made no difference to their state of erection and two found that it actually enhanced erection. One of the latter explained that since his early teens he would get slight erections when feeling anxious.

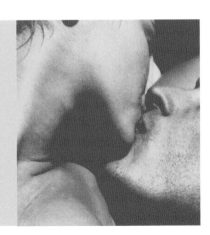

SEX AND THE PRESIDENCY

A further theory about ex-President Clinton is that he is a man who associates feeling better with sexual release. When you think about the major stresses he had to juggle daily, his behaviour, unsuitable though it was for a president, does not, in this light, seem so surprising. He is an illustration of how muddled the states of anxiety and sexuality can become!

How anxiety affects sex It's the muddle that is worth concentrating on because, if ever there were an example of how reactions can run riot, it is in the range of responses that human beings experience sexually as a result of anxiety. According to Bancroft anxiety can:

- Interfere with sexual response, either speeding it up or slowing it down;
- Interfere with thought processes that would lead to a reasoned assessment of the situation;
- Be avoided by inhibiting some sexual responses;
- Be a reaction to sexual failure;
- Facilitate sexual response.

I don't list these possibilities to confuse you although you could be forgiven if they do, but to illustrate how different our various responses can be to the same emotion. Individuals, possessing different ideas about life, will feel these enormously varied responses.

Anger

There is also evidence that anger can sometimes fuel and facilitate sexual response rather than inhibit it.

How anger affects sex Anger works in several interesting ways, one of which is that it may improve sexual response. Yet some people cannot feel both angry and sexy at the same time. Perhaps a degree of anger is stimulating, but if it increases and resentment evolves, then this further degree of rage will erode sex. Avoidance or rejection of sexual activity may be a way of expressing anger. Rape, of course, is a vicious method of expressing anger.

Don't automatically assume that powerful negative
emotions mean you can't be sexual.
Adjust your ideas and find out.

Elation and Depression

Elation and depression are at opposite ends of the emotional spectrum and each can influence what goes on between the sheets. Gina's story, below, illustrates this very well. You may get the impression when you read it that Gina was a young, beautiful woman with a perfect shape – the kind of ideal we are told men really go for. It could come as a surprise, therefore, to learn that Gina was overweight, middle-aged and not particularly stylish. Which is my point.

You are as attractive as you feel you are.
You can be just about anything you want if you believe strongly.
You are what you believe.

GINA'S STORY

Gina suffered from bipolar disorder, the condition that used to be called manic depression. On the occasions when she felt manic, she felt sexually empowered. Her drive was high, her energy boundless, and her confidence endless. With these as a basis of physical and emotional wellbeing, she believed she could do virtually anything sexual – and she did; no holds barred. She swung. She enjoyed multiple partners. She climaxed easily and quickly. She believed she was powerfully attractive and acted as if she were. Men flocked around her.

As the disorder gained ground, Gina experienced depression more often than elation. With depression, everything shut down. Her energy disappeared, her sex drive shrank, and her self-belief vanished. Instead of getting out and chasing lovers, she could hardly stir from her room.

Gina's story is an extreme one. I recount it to provide a dramatic illustration of how mood can affect both sexuality and self-belief. It is a curse to suffer from intense mood swings. Nobody would wish it. But many of us might want to gain some of Gina's self-belief (experienced when manic). An important point about her story is the fact that her body chemistry affected her personal beliefs. The medical profession today is concentrating hard on that connection between mind and body, not only for sufferers from bipolar disorder but for all the rest of us who at some time or other fall prey to depression.

How depression affects sex drive

Depression

- Lowers sexual desire;
- Impairs erection in men;
- Impairs erection and lubrication in women;
- Makes orgasm difficult to reach.

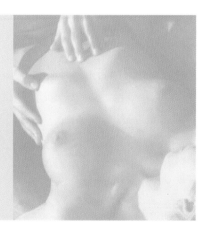

TESTOSTERONE AND SEX DRIVE

It is now widely suspected that testosterone is responsible for sex drive in women as well as in men. So if depression hits men in their libido, there's every reason to think it will do the same for women. Supplementation with the hormone allows men to feel reassuringly sexual while women who are given testosterone report much stronger sexual feelings.

Impaired sleep erections in men (which are found in cases of low sexual desire and low free-ranging testosterone), are also found in depressive illness. New antidepressants are constantly being developed to combat various forms of depression. These raise the mood and usually allow sexual desire and arousal to return.

Mood Treatments

When we get really depressed most of us feel desperate enough to opt for anti-depressants or talking treatments or, ideally, a combination of both. But one problem is that often we don't recognize we have become depressed.

We assume that feeling continually grim is normal. It isn't. To alleviate this kind of misery we need to do two things. The first is to halt the chemical aspect of depression in its tracks. This usually needs to be done first because without putting a brake on the depression, it is hard to concentrate on any kind of talking treatment. And when it is hard to concentrate, it is very hard indeed to do any of the work needed to sort out our heads. Once the head feels clearer, thanks to anti-depressants, we get fit enough to tackle whatever caused the difficulty in the first place.

The moral of this story is: if your sex life has flown out of the window, stop and think about your mood. If you are depressed, you may need an antidepressant to stop the flow of misery and let you feel generally better. If you have any kind of hormone impairment, first of all you need to find out what your body chemicals are doing. When you have done so (by paying a visit to the doctor), you then need to think about hormone readjustment, or, in cases of older men and women, hormone replacement.

Drugs

What? Take drugs? Without being ill? A terrible idea, I hear you cry. Stop for a minute and think. If we go back to the theory of memes, an idea is something that can mutate. Why should your idea that taking drugs is harmful still hold true today? Wouldn't it be worth, at least, reassessing the situation?

Drugs have traditionally been held to be a bad idea because they might be addictive and/or possess dangerous side-effects. These beliefs were based on a historic reality. The early development of drugs has been a hazardous process. But we have been developing them now for well over a century. Many of the prejudices we feel today were sensible ones 20 years ago. But things move fast in biochemical research and, before we dismiss an important life choice out of hand we ought at least to get ourselves up to scratch.

These days we don't hesitate to turn to drugs when we feel that there is just cause. We hail them as life savers when we:

- Recover from cancer;
- Don't die from gangrene;
- Mitigate the ravages of arthritis;
- Survive common flu instead of dying from the high temperatures it creates.

Yet we still believe we should not resort to drugs without dire cause. So far it is only life-saving situations or intense pain that allow us to feel drug-taking is OK. Yet now that drugs that affect well-being are becoming honed and statistically safe, couldn't we begin to change our beliefs – just a tad? One reason why it's important to keep your mind open is because new information is constantly being fed into it. Just as a computer shifts its conclusions slightly every time new data is entered, so, too, do our brains. If you add a couple of new facts to the hotchpotch of beliefs presently jostling for space, you must gain a different picture – mustn't you?

Why should we have to feel seriously ill just to improve our quality of life? One of the golden rules of assertion training is that it is all right to change your mind because doing so is a sign of maturity.

Drugs that improve sex Today there are drugs that can improve our body chemistry so that we no longer experience depression and, as a result, can gain a rejuvenation of sexual desire.

Drugs can also moderate both the excitor and the inhibitor centres in the brain, so that we can turn on or turn off when previously this had been difficult. They can also dampen down anxiety so that we can function well enough to improve our relationship with the man or woman we love and subsequently perform well in the bedroom.

Finally, drugs can prolong and assist erection.

Testosterone, which has been regarded with suspicion for 50 years, has come of age. Research shows that regular testosterone use for men over a period of almost 60 years, far from causing health problems, safeguards against arteriosclerosis and allows men to feel energetic, good-tempered and reassuringly sexual. There is no equivalent long-term information about women yet, but individual reports of women using testosterone gel rubbed into the skin, indicate that these women feel stronger, have more energy, enjoy increased sexual sensation in the genitals and achieve orgasm with greater ease. Unless some totally unexpected finding (which hasn't happened with men) demonstrates a disastrous side-effect, can you think of any reason why women should not feel all these life-affirming sensations for as long as is possible? I can't.

Drugs that improve life   There is also a powerful belief (another meme) that the forth-coming century will see a greater acceptance of miracle drugs, which prevent emotional suffering much as chemotherapy and penicillin have prevented physical suffering in the past. For drugs have moved into a second phase. Now that we know we can cure or at least halt the progression of serious illness the next step is to not only deal with the life or death situations but to look at the quality of life as well.

We only have one life to live. And it is a short one. If you knew that you were going to spend two-thirds of it crippled with arthritis wouldn't you gladly opt for a drug that would guarantee you pain-free flexible joints even if you did have to take one of those pills every day for the rest of your life? Why shouldn't we adopt the same attitude towards substances that improve the way we experience our sex life?

There is a lot of evidence to show that men and women,
given half a chance, are happy to be sexy for ever.

Sixty-year-old women these days still only look around 40, compared to previous genera-tions. That's thanks to hormone replacement. And, far from risking your life through taking hormone therapy, the opposite is probably true. You are likely to prolong it.

Overcoming drug-related anxieties   Why am I bothering to bang on in this way if you are prejudiced against taking drugs? Because I hope to start you thinking differently about them. I hope that, through the information presented here, fresh ideas will allow you to process the pill-gulping decision with more real choice. If you block out information because of prejudice, you do not possess real choice. I can't bear important options to be missed because your decisions are based on outdated facts from 50 years ago.

So what about those beliefs (or prejudices) that we started off with? Let's go over them.

Addiction
Yes, we may find we can't manage very well without the drugs, once we've started, but this isn't surprising since we weren't managing very well before we started taking them. In fact,

OESTROGEN EQUALS WELLBEING

Oestrogen makes you feel well. It also guards against osteoporosis and heart disease – two killers in old age. The evidence linking oestrogen with cancer continues to be debatable as studies show both positive and negative results. If you are taking oestrogen though, you are more likely to receive regular gynaecological check-ups so that if there are any precancerous changes they will be spotted early and dealt with, giving a high chance of living on for years. The saddest story in my own history is of one of my school friends who died at the age of 42 because she had never, in her entire life, had a cervical smear.

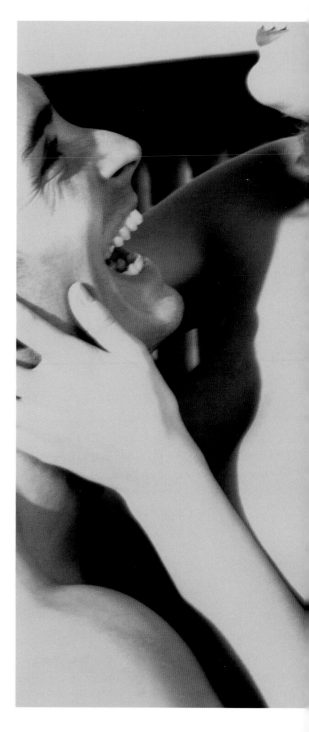

that is why we started taking them. What the drugs increasingly do is fulfill a function that our body, for reasons of its own, has stopped doing.

I suspect most of us wouldn't think twice about using a bionic leg aid if our real leg could hardly function – particularly if we were given the opportunity of receiving a prosthetic leg that looked exactly like the real one. And if the real leg eventually chose to not walk at all, well, there would be no argument, would there? We would be grateful for the bionic system and might even find that certain walking and running abilities functioned better than the original. Drugs go one better. With drugs there is the possibility that their use may kickstart the original system into

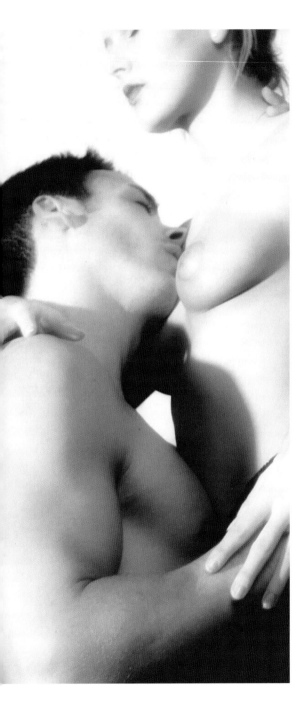

functioning again so that we don't have to prolong their use.

In the past we have only considered using drugs as a temporary measure to get us better. In the future, we may choose to use drugs long-term to improve our quality of life. The fact that thousands of men opted for Viagra when it first hit the market shows we are already moving in this direction. And if women thought that a female version of this little blue pill would guarantee them a good sexual response (including an orgasm), it is highly likely that women, too, would start popping pills with far greater ease. Some psychiatrists already believe that long-term usage of certain medications would improve the quality of life for great swathes of the population.

Dangerous side-effects

If you heard that a particular pill would make you turn blue, then, if you were sensible, you would research it before rejecting it out of hand. If you subsequently discovered that it is only people with blood group B-positive who turn blue, and you know you are not B-positive, then, on the face of it, there wouldn't seem to be much reason for holding back from improving your life.

My point is you need to know as much as possible about all side-effects of any pill before swallowing it. But you can only make a responsible decision when all the facts are marshalled before you. So one duty of anyone wanting to improve his or her love life chemically is to thoroughly research the consequences of his or her choice first. But if, on having done so, the evidence is that you will be able to tolerate the drug, please don't then dismiss it out of prejudice.

Many of the new substances used in hormone replacement therapy are now formulated as gels or creams to be rubbed into the skin rather than taken orally. The great advantage of this method is that the substance in question gets directly into the bloodstream without having to be processed by the stomach and liver. Much of the damage done to the human system through pill-swallowing is as a result of damage to the liver. Now we know to avoid this method.

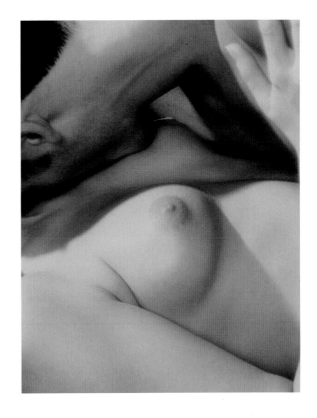

So, before dismissing the notion of drug-taking out of hand, please research the substance in question. Read the accompanying notes that arrive with it. Look it up in medical dictionaries, go to the internet and feed details of the drug into as many search engines as you can muster. If what you get back is a catalogue of disasters, don't go near it. But if the reviews are favourable, please consider it. Especially if it comes in gel or cream form.

Men and women flock to 'natural' cures in their thousands. Health food shops sell tons of natural supplements, vitamins and creams. Aromatherapy has become big business with major chain stores selling aromatic oils. One out of four people reading this book is likely to have experienced some kind of massage using aromatic oil (or even baby oil) – and lived to tell the tale. Did you know that your skin will absorb any substance put on it? That those 'natural cures' still bring about physical and chemical changes? Most of us have been subjecting our bodies to these 'natural' chemical changes for years now yet continue to function just fine.

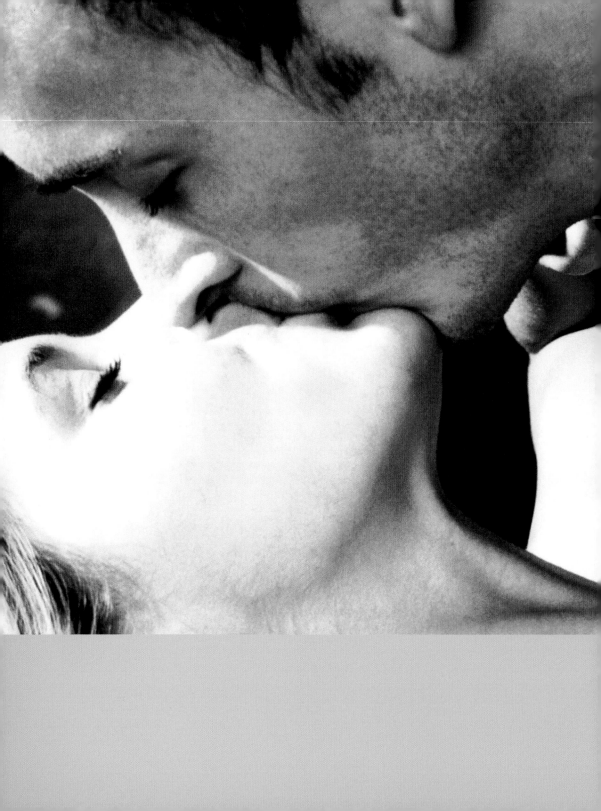

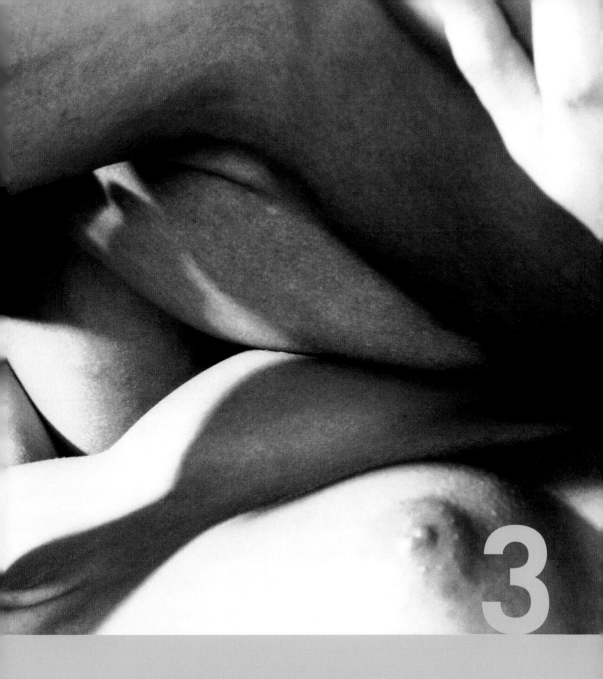

3

Turning Your Sex Life Around

Mind Over Matter

'An erection cannot be willed.' This is a common belief, which on the face of it appears to be true. Men usually can't produce erections for every circumstance or at least we think this to be the case. But... this is only partly true. The evidence shows something else. Surveys, clinical studies and laboratory experiments have demonstrated that many men (and women) can produce genital responses at will, by thinking sexual thoughts or unrolling sexual fantasies in their heads. And they can do this in front of other people (i.e. in front of laboratory technicians). The same experiments have also shown that people can distract themselves from becoming turned on by thinking non-sexual thoughts.

The use of erotic films and of fantasy got the sexual systems of these men and women under observation up and firing and resulting in all kinds of delicious sensory reactions in circumstances where most of us would have thought that feeling sexy was a non-starter.

On the strength of this information, let me float an idea.
Unless there is something physically wrong
– a possibility which can be established by medical tests –
you will be able to function sexually.

The only reason you won't be functioning sexually, therefore, is because you don't want to. In other words, even if you are not consciously doing this, you are unconsciously choosing not to be sexual. Your lack of desire or erection might feel like a problem, it certainly may be creating a problem. But it is your choice.

In this event, you might like to think about your needs for making such a choice. What is such a choice letting you do that in other circumstances you couldn't or wouldn't? What benefits and/or advantages does it bring?

Alternatively, you might like to change that choice now that you know you have made it. Or you might like to think about changing your relationship. How you make such decisions depends on the ideas you bring to the problem situation and then the ways in which you choose to reframe them. So let's contemplate reframing. In therapeutic circles this is titled cognitive feedback.

Sexual Attitude Restructuring

No, I didn't make this phrase up. Sexual attitude restructuring (SAR) is an idea pioneered by the Reverend Ted McIlvenna of the Glide Foundation and of the Institute for the Advanced Study of Human Sexuality in San Francisco. It is a process that mature students willingly undergo before studying for their qualifications in Human Sexuality. The Institute is the only organization in the United States licensed to award a degree in Human Sexuality. It has remained the only institution to do so for the past 25 years.

In order to approach the subject of human sexuality with a non-judgemental approach, Institute officials (these include Wardell Pomeroy, one of the co-authors of the famous Kinsey report) realized that contemporary men and women are thoroughly handicapped by the sex information they have already picked up in the world and therefore need retraining. How could an individual expect to make important decisions about sex, if he or she is inculcated with prejudice and misbelief?

At the very least, a SAR training aims to provide up-to-date accurate information about human sexual behaviour. At the most, it hopes to clear the mind of misinformation and prejudice so that the students can go on to make balanced and reasonable decisions about their own sex lives and about men and women who are likely to be their counselling clients. Most SAR students are already in the helping professions while more are beginning their therapy training. Students are typically sex therapists, counsellors, social workers, teachers, psychiatrists, psychologists and family doctors.

The Role of Sex Films

The SAR weekend consists of a blitz of sex education films interspersed with discussions on the particular sexual subject that has been featured. Over the weekend, the students view around 60 separate films; these are often screened three at a time. The films are on just about every aspect of sexuality you might care to name. And they are not movies acted out by actors and actresses. They are films of real people – documentary style – showing their real sex patterns, the real ways in which they actually make love, have sex, fuck.

In 1964, Ted McIlvenna, a young Methodist minister, came to work at the Methodist Glide Foundation to work with young people. While doing so, he became acutely aware of how alienated young homosexuals were from the church and of how damaged they became when they did try to seek advice from clergy, physicians or others, often because of the

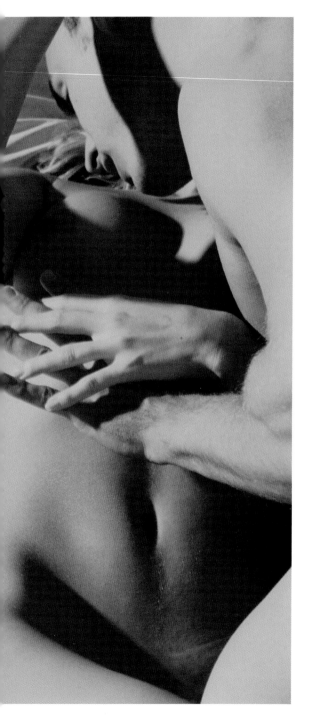

personal hang-ups of these so called 'helpers'. Realizing that you can't understand homosexuality without understanding human sexuality, McIlvenna and his team, began experimenting with a new and exceedingly controversial system that would help professionals gain a broader view of sex so that, in turn, they could truly help people in distress.

He and Laird Sutton, a young film-maker, asked permission of certain couples, often students, that they might film them making love. When the films were edited, the students were promised that the movies would be shown to them first so that they could comment on whether or not they felt the footage to be a fair portrayal of their sexual behaviour. If the films were considered inaccurate, the couples could veto them. Over the years, the Glide Foundation built up a bank of sex films unlike any other, virtually constituting a thesis in themselves. Here, on the screen, could be seen a unique archive of real sexual behaviour.

It sounds easy described on paper, almost 40 years after the inception of such an extraordinary project. But making such films while maintaining any kind of dignified and respected status quo was not easy. It says a great deal about Ted McIlvenna's giant personality that he managed to make it look effortless when it can have been nothing of the sort. His was a truly original and innovative inspiration.

The films and the ensuing discussion became the basis for the training scheme, which 11 years later, became the foundation of the institute.

An Open Attitude Towards Sex

By the time a SAR weekend is over, everyone attending can talk about any aspect of sex without turning a hair. This means that it provides wonderful food for mending your own relationship – it also means that when a client comes to you, finding it exceedingly hard to talk about a subject so traditionally secret, he or she responds to your comfort with the subject. Clients grow comfortable themselves. How many people do you know who have tried to talk about sexual difficulties with a doctor or counsellor only to come to an abrupt halt because the helper in question was so embarrassed by the subject?

You might expect that some participants of such an overt training system would be dissatisfied with the extraordinarily intimate nature of the subject matter. McIlvenna and his staff have been sensibly careful to take notice of all feedback. Statistics show that 96 per cent of participants find the SAR very helpful both personally and professionally. Three per cent are not sure and one per cent find it of no value. I doubt if many other training establishments show such remarkable results.

If Ted McIlvenna himself had not been able to shed traditional thoughts and prejudices about sex, his extraordinary training institution would never have produced the thousands of graduates that it has done over the years. Almost every sex educator in the United States and Canada and many more in the United Kingdom have experienced the SAR programme – not just the weekend course specifically referred to here but the full-time training that results in several different types of degree award.

Turning Your Own Sex Life Around

The SAR system doesn't only teach you to be a better counsellor, it also makes a major difference to how you handle your own sex life. I quote here a paragraph from the *SAR Guide* (1975).

'For a long time, we have been aware that persons attending the Forum's basic introductory course have in great measure solved a lot of their sexual problems. This has also been observed by others in the sex field. Our conclusion is that most of so-called sexual dysfunction results from lack of knowledge. Where there is no physical problem involved, most persons find they can change their patterns simply through a change of attitude and actions, whether or not they have had difficulty in achieving orgasm, controlling premature ejaculation or maintaining potency.'

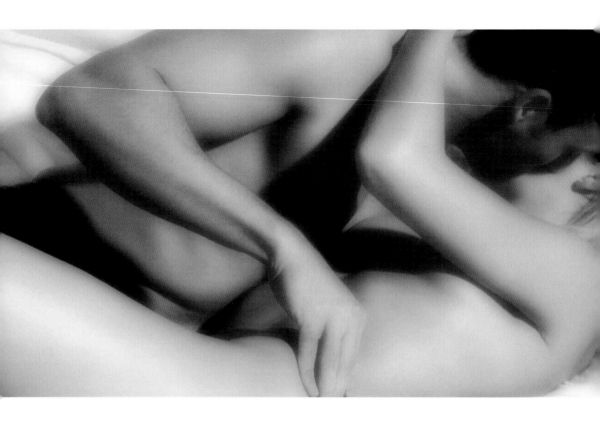

Over the next few pages, I am going to outline a few exercises based on these methods in the hope that they will allow you, too, to develop a sense of familiarity with sex so that it is not so loaded a subject. I do this in the hope that once sex stops being quite such a big deal, you will find you are able to think differently about it and to make decisions about sex in a less stressed manner. Naturally I can only outline a few of the ideas that the Institute teaches in great detail. And so that I don't poach the methods, which are the Institute's hallmark, what you see in these pages is entirely my own version of attitude restructuring. If you want to enrol for the real SAR you will find the address and telephone number of the Institute in the appendix on page 160.

I also hope I've made a good enough case in the two preceding sections for offering here a system which allows you to look at sex differently via a process of getting familiar with deeply intimate sex acts.

Changing Sexual Prejudices

If you want to get the most out of this programme, I suggest you work through it sequentially. You need to read straight through the entire collection of visualizations that follows, stopping only briefly in between visualizations to think through your feelings or, if you are with a friend or in a group, to talk through thoroughly what you have just viewed. If you break off halfway through the series and come back to it later, you won't get the same impact and the programme won't work. The object of the programme is to get much more comfortable with sexual intimacy until you reach a point where you can accept a variety of sex acts without bringing a judgementally laden attitude to them. You don't have to change one iota regarding your own sex life if you don't want to. Nothing is imperative. But it would be good to think that you might change your acceptance of others.

Know Yourself

In order to change your sexual attitudes, you need to know what they consist of first. These questions allow you to take yourself through a type of sex life history. Please answer the questions sequentially.

The idea behind the questions is not that there are any right or wrong answers, but that by replying truthfully, you may get to know yourself rather better than before. Even though we experience certain sexual events, we don't always put them together and make any kind of pattern from them. The answers here will help gain insight into your own particular sexual preferences.

Patterns that can emerge are:

- An open enjoyment of sexuality – usually where the parental example has been a positive one and where discussion about sex in the family has been open;
- A difficulty in sexual enjoyment – often where the parental example has been negative and sex a taboo subject in the family. Very strong religious beliefs can also adversely affect sexual enjoyment;
- A difficulty in relating sexually to one particular person but not to others;
- A lack of relating sexually;
- An abundance of relating sexually that may get you into trouble.

WHAT PATTERNS CAN YOU SEE FOR YOURSELF?

- What ideas about sex did you gain from your parents?
- What kind of a loving or non-loving example did your parents set?
- If you could take a guess at the quality of your parents' sex life, how would you rate it? Excellent, good, fair, poor, non-existent?
- Who or what else did you learn about sex from? Siblings, school friends, other friends, teachers, magazines?
- At what age did you discover masturbation? And in what circumstances? How did you feel about it?
- Have you ever fantasized? And if you have, how old were you when this first happened?
- Did you ever experience sex (wet) dreams as a child?
- Do your religious beliefs play any part in your experience of sexuality?
- How important is sexual pleasure to you?
- Have you experienced orgasm?
- Do you feel comfortable in talking about sex?
- How old were you when you had your first sex experience?
- Did this feel good or poor?
- In what physical circumstances did you first have sex (i.e. bed, car, field)?
- What has been your best sex experience?
- What has been your worst sex experience?
- How many sex partners have you had during your lifetime?
- Have you taken part in any group sex activity (i.e. threesome, couples, swinging, etc.)?
- Have you ever been raped or forced into having sex against your will?
- How do you feel about sex right now?
- Have you had sexual relationships outside your main relationship?
- How do you feel about these?
- What have you learned sexually from your long-term relationship(s)?

Know Your Partner

It's sensible to ask your partner to answer these questions, too, and then to share the results. If you are in the early days of relating, this probably won't be difficult. If you have been together for a while, it may get more sensitive. If you don't want to know about possible infidelities, leave out this section. By sharing information you can compare and pinpoint areas that you have in common and areas where you seem different. It makes sense to build on the shared aspects and work on opening up to the different ones.

What Do You Want to Achieve From Your Sex Life?

You probably wouldn't be reading this book if there wasn't something you specially wanted from it – even if it is just to wallow in sexual ideas.

You might want to:
- Know yourself better;
- Widen your sexual horizons;
- Improve your sexual expertise;
- Feel sexy more of the time;
- Improve the sex side of your relationship;
- Feel all right about doing something sexually daring?

What it is that you want? Try to get a handle on what you might be looking for at this special moment in time.

Keeping A Sexual Diary

Even if you can't write for toffee try keeping a sexual diary. Nobody else is going to read it except for you. The value of this is that when you look back over a couple of months you can see patterns emerge in your sex life. Sometimes those patterns contradict what you have previously believed about yourself. One man had considered himself to be sexually inadequate, (in part because he was constantly undermined by his father). But on re-reading his diary, he discovered himself to be highly sexual. He both satisfied his girlfriend and himself with intercourse and, on the evenings he didn't see her, he always masturbated to orgasm. There was nothing wrong with his sex drive or his expression of it. But it took the proof, in black and white, to change his idea about himself.

• PICTURE YOUR FAVOURITE MOVIE STAR. HE (OR SHE) IS STANDING FACING THE CAMERA HOLDING A LONG LIST. IT'S SO LONG THAT IT LOOKS LIKE A REEL OF LAVATORY PAPER. THIS IS A LIST OF SEX WORDS, THE STAR ANNOUNCES. HE OR SHE IS GOING TO READ THEM OUT LOUD. AND READ THEM OUT LOUD, HE OR SHE DOES. HERE'S WHAT IS READ:

POKE

FUCK

ARSE, CUNT, WANK

GASP

CUM, PRICK, PULL

LICK, SUCK, RIM

THRUST

ARSE-FUCK

BITCH, WHORE

GROAN, SWEAT, SEEP

DRIP, BALLS, TESTICLES

FINGER-FUCK

SCREW   SPILL

JACK-OFF

                    DRIBBLE

SLIP, SQUINT

- NOW READ THESE OUT LOUD YOURSELF — IN A LOUD VOICE.
NOW DO IT AGAIN. HOW ARE YOU FEELING? STOPPED IN YOUR TRACKS?
FAINTLY SHOCKED? STIMULATED? TURNED ON? CARRY ON READING THE
LIST OVER AND OVER AGAIN. EVENTUALLY YOU WILL FIND THAT THE
WORDS HAVE LESS IMPACT. CARRY ON SOME MORE. EVENTUALLY THE
WORDS BECOME SIMPLY ... WORDS.

Reading About Sex

Books about sex as well as sexy books can provide several vital functions. You may get to feel much hornier from reading about sex which, if you worry about not turning on too easily, can be vastly reassuring. Books can give you a rich sex life when your actual sex life presently feels empty. You also can learn a lot from them about both sex and relationships – never a bad thing.

So please pay no attention to the critics who rubbish sexual reading material. If you want to read it, go right ahead. One safeguard here: if you are in a relationship where the other person may feel threatened by your reading sex books, please either explain that you are doing this as part of an educational course and invite him or her to join you. Or, if you truly feel this wouldn't work, protect the other person by ensuring he or she doesn't know much about your reading matter.

Any time you meet with someone else's opposition to something that concerns sex, remind yourself that this opposition is based on one particular set of ideas. And that the reason you are clashing is because you hold a different set of ideas. You are entitled to your different ideas – just as he or she is. This is not a license to upset or hurt others but it is a permission to feel all right about yourself. Just remind yourself you are experiencing a struggle between memes!

Sexual Practise

One way of finding out just what your prejudices consist of is to embark on a series of daring visualisations (pages 56–79). Read them through quickly. When you finish, stop and examine your feelings As you embark on each of the visualizations ask yourself how you feel about each particular scene. Do you experience:

- Violent loathing?
- Dislike?
- Nothing much?
- A pleasing tinge of interest?
- Acute turn-on?

Each of these reactions gives you a good idea of what you do or don't feel comfortable with. Pinpoint your prejudices.

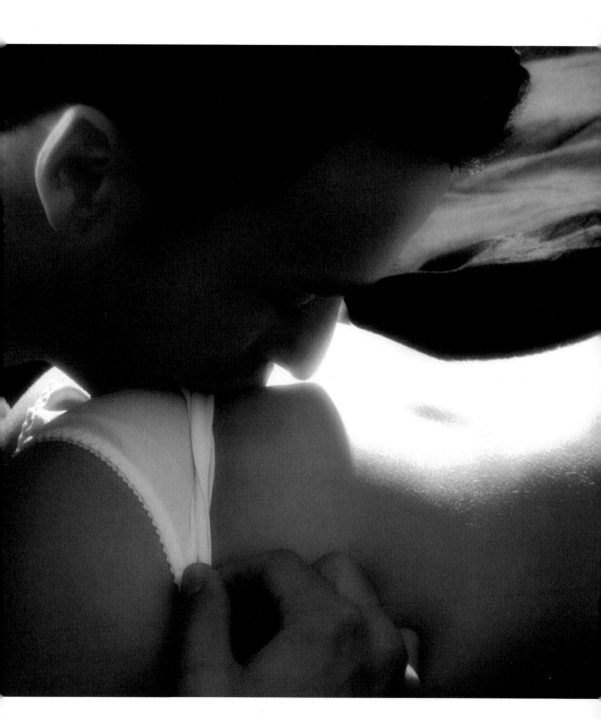

Cute Cartoon Hamsters

Hammy and Honey are cute hamsters. They are just youngsters, jumping about in the garden, enjoying the rough-and-tumble of childish games. They box and scrabble and roll around, ending up as far away as the long grass. They possess very silly faces that register surprise every time they fetch up against a rock, a plant or each other. As they jump up and down on top of each other, their weight (hamsters are hefty little creatures) fair knock the breath out of each other. You'd think they'd get used to this but no, every time it happens, they look really puzzled. You can't help laughing. Every jump gets a bit more silly, with the creatures landing on each other in a variety of very silly positions, sideways, lengthways, upside down, sprawled across each other so that every position gets funnier. When the hamsters start jumping a bit more rhythmically, and they (and you) realize that by sheer accident they appear to be having sex, the surprise on their faces is priceless. You all roar with laughter. The transition from fun to sex has been seamless. The hamsters are innocent and the sex is just a part of playing.

♥ *How do you feel? You have just watched sex on the screen of your imagination. Try going over the scene again.*

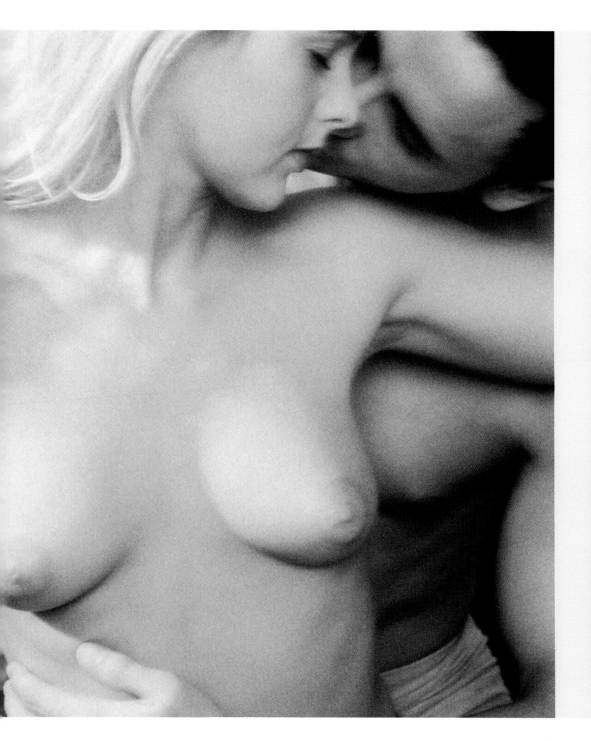

Young Lovers

Switch your mind to a pair of young lovers. These are real lovers – not actors, an ordinary girl and boy – probably students at college. They are lying on his bed in the middle of the afternoon. You can tell this is real because the room is a mess and they haven't cleared up the dishes from lunchtime. They are fully clothed and kissing passionately. You can tell this isn't the first time they have made love because they look comfortable with each other. They are lying close, running their hands all over each other's bodies and delving underneath each other's clothes. At some point they stop caressing and separately take their clothes off. They lie down again and carry on kissing and caressing. You see his hand disappear between her legs and guess from the regular movements that he is rhythmically stroking her clitoris. She stretches and purrs in approval, then settles to become almost motionless as she concentrates on the sensation that is building inside her. 'Stop,' she says, 'come inside me' and she urges him to climb over her and insert his penis into her vagina. She pushes her pelvis up towards him and you can just see the in/out of his thrusting. If you look at her face you realize that she has gone into a world of the interior, her eyes are glazed, her attention far away, where only sexual feelings matter. 'Help me a little,' she asks. He accordingly shifts one thigh and inserts his hand between their bodies. As he continues to thrust, his arm drums to the rhythm he is whipping up on her clitoris. Suddenly she starts to come, with her body shuddering and her head thrown back, rapid breathing huffs from her mouth. When she hits the high point of coming, she screams. And as long as she goes on screaming her young lover does not let up. He thrusts and fingers with great energy. He drives on and forward, on and forward. It is only when he is quite clear her climax is over that he withdraws his hand, closes his eyes and focuses on his own thrusting. When he climaxes, he does so in a quick series of spurts and hard gasps. 'Oh,' he cries, short and sharp, then collapses on her in a happy heap. She folds her arms around him and gathers his limp body in to hers.

Does this scene disturb you? Does it feel wrong to read it? Forbidden? Upsetting? If you are not sure of your emotion, read the description again.

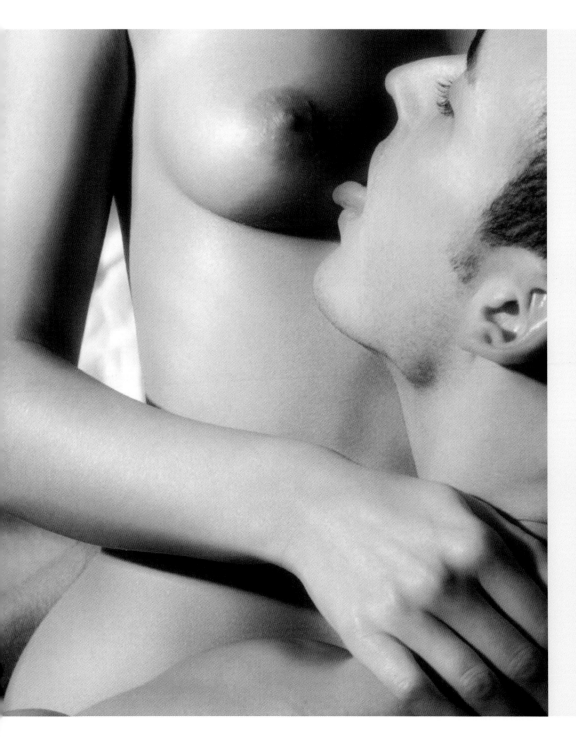

Male Masturbation

Let your imagination take you to the far side of a bedroom. You are hidden, but from your hiding place you can see a man lying on the bed. You know that this is for real, this is not an actor from a porn movie in spite of his being young and handsome. This man is moving about a lot, in fact, from your distance, it looks as if he is feeling uncomfortable. You zoom your viewing in closer and see that the reason he is moving is because he is masturbating. But this is not some still and passive jerk-off. This young male is moving his entire body as he moves his cock. He kneels up to manipulate his penis, one hand doing the task while the other roams all over his body, stroking, pushing, kneading. He bends over and continues to pull on his penis as he leans on all fours. As he increases the rhythm of his cock he starts to move his entire body, backwards and forwards, into his hand. He literally undulates in and out of wanking on all fours. Now he gets off the bed and leaning against it upright, juts his cock hard out into the room as he pounds away, his hips jerking his penis into and out of the cylinder that is his hand. He literally dances across the room moving that penis in and out of his grasp until with a great explosion he comes while he is arched up on one foot in a kind of arabesque.

You may think this sounds an unlikely visualization of male masturbation but it is based on one of the Glide Foundation films and it is real. The young man filmed was a ballet dancer and put his entire body into self-satisfaction. How did you feel about it? Is there another way in which you would prefer to see a male masturbating? One that feels more realistic to you? Here is an alternative.

A man is washing himself in the bath. After he has efficiently soaped his body, he leans back to rest in the suds and relax. Slowly, lazily, his hands creep down to his genitals. While one hand holds his penis at the base, the other lazily pulls up on the penis several times until his penis stands by itself. Still holding it at the base he uses the other hand, palm down, to rub around and over the head of the penis, lemon squeezer style. He's in no particular hurry. And he is very deliberate. Next he pulls up with the underneath hand while continuing to rub and circle on the head, then pushes down again with the lower hand.

He's got two very precise actions going on simultaneously with his busy hands. The rest of his body is still and quite soon straining forwards. Now he's not so slow. He is much more excited and his two hands get rough. He's gripping his cock and moving hard and fast, very fast. Surely that must hurt, you think, as you see him pumping in a blur of speed. Now his body is keeping time with the action, chucking a little bathwater over the side. It's so fast you know he's out of control. It would be hard to stop now. Suddenly and quickly his penis erupts into an arc of pure fluid jetting towards the end of the tub. As it does so he subsides groaning into the by-now tepid water.

Does this description feel more realistic? More like what you might expect? And what did you feel? Shock? Disgust? Pleasure? Or acceptance? Don't get sidetracked into thinking this is the right way to masturbate. Any way is the right way. There is no one typical way.

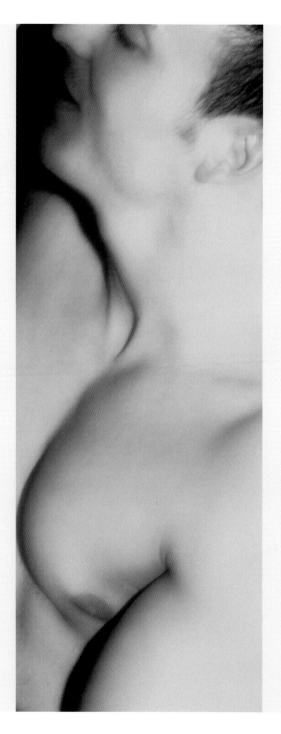

Female Masturbation

She is 30-something and plump. She steps into the shower and soaps herself luxuriously, creating a lot of foam which she rinses off while playing the pinpoints of water from the shower head across her skin for a long while. As she steps out of the shower cubicle she helps herself to a warm towel from the towel rail and wanders into the bedroom comfortably drying herself. She strips the top sheets from the bed and places a dry towel over the bottom sheet. She gathers up a box of tissues and some massage oil, which she places on the bedside table. Now she makes herself comfortable, leaning back onto a circle of cushions. Using some of the oil she rubs it all over her body and especially around her breasts. She squeezes and kneads her breasts and evidently gets a lot of pleasure from doing this because you can see her noticeably relax and sink back. In fact, she so enjoys this that it takes a while before she moves her hands down to her genitals. When she does so she holds her labia open with her left hand so that the pink interior is exposed. Then with one finger of the right hand she gently, oh so gently, starts to rub on her clitoris. As she gets more excited she pulls her labia up hard and arches her back a little. Dissatisfied with this, she shifts her left hand underneath her left thigh and reaching up with it from underneath, puts a finger into her vagina and pulls downwards. She gasps almost immediately, such is the easy turn-on this gives her, and accelerates her twirling and rubbing of the clitoris with the right hand. Now she jerks her pelvis towards that thrusting top finger, and each time she does so gasps as she pulls against that constraining bottom finger. Her head falls backwards, her mouth opens a little and her hips jerk convulsively as she comes again and again. She doesn't stop the stimulation though – she goes right on and on rubbing and climaxing many times until finally the climaxes die away. Awkwardly, heavily, she removes the arm that has become trapped underneath her satisfied pelvis, with an effort heaves her legs together and lies panting as if getting her breath back.

♥ *This is the real masturbation pattern of a real woman. Did it hold any surprises for you? Did you feel embarrassed by viewing it? Was it like anything you have seen or experienced? Try re-running it again to check out your reactions. Now try this alternative.*

Visualize the same woman, stepping into the same shower. She goes through the same bathing routine, rubbing herself with foaming soap and luxuriously showering it off with the carefully directed shower head. Only this time she doesn't get out of the shower because she's become far too interested in the tiny pin prick of sensuality that the shower water evokes on her genitals. She holds the showerhead at crotch position and squats slightly so that her legs are as wide as they can be without letting her fall over. The shower plays upon her labia, the outer end of her vagina and her clitoris. But presumably the sensation isn't strong enough for she does two things. The first is she readjusts the flow of water so that it spurts out much harder and the second is that she holds her labia open with two fingers so that the water cannot miss her clitoris. After a while, she stands very still and shuts her eyes. You sense that the drumming of the tiny water jets is stirring up an acute sensation. Suddenly she staggers and puts out a hand to avoid slipping, but carries on drumming the jets at her clitoris. Almost immediately, she

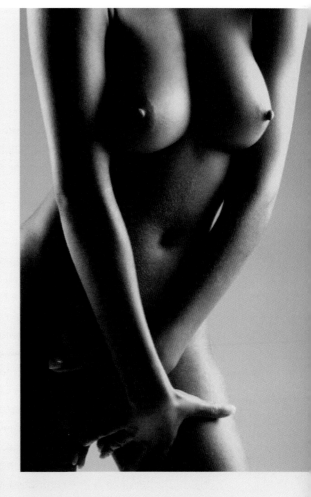

starts jerking her pelvis forward into the spray. 'Oh,' she says softly, "Oh.' It doesn't last for long but it was there. Now she feels so overcome that she turns the shower off, sits on the shower tray and clasps and presses her hands between her legs. 'Wow,' she says, 'Wow.'

You have just visualized a completely different masturbation pattern to the one described before and yet it has been experienced by the same woman. There are many different ways of climaxing. Human beings are creative. If you have masturbated, how many different ways have you ever done it? If you haven't experimented, perhaps after this you might like to try?

Letting Go During Sex

A couple in their mid-30s settle down on a mattress in the living room. The mattress is covered with a sheepskin rug, there are plants dotted about the room and you can tell it's afternoon from the angle of the sun shining through the curtain-free windows. You take a quick peer through the window and discover, with relief, that it is on the second storey and not overlooked. 'I'm giving you a treat today,' says the woman and produces a bottle of massage oil. She oils and greases his body and works on it for a good 10 minutes, firmly pushing and gliding her hands about his back. When she turns him over to cover his front you see that he has an erection. She laughs and massages his front, eventually including the erection in the massage. When you take a closer look at the man's face you see his eyes are open and glazed with pleasure. You also see that his expression is changing; he is deciding to change the action. 'Come here,' he says and pulls his woman's naked body on to his. She slides and swims across the oil slick that soon coats them both. His erection is standing up harder than ever. Next, he starts to press her down towards that erection so that it catches between her legs and then comes free again as he slides her up towards his chest. Up and down until they are both panting and flushed. 'It's so hot in here,' she gasps, raising a hand to wipe the perspiration from her face. 'That's how I like it,' he says abruptly and catching her arms turns her sideways onto the mattress. Without waiting for her reaction he puts his large hand between her legs and begins to rub his entire fist up and down. And his movements are hard. At one stage he stops, spits onto his hand and rubs the spit into her genitals. She is gasping with sharp intakes of breath now as he shoves that hand backwards and forwards, scraping across her labia and grinding across her clitoris, backwards and forwards. He heaves her up onto all fours, moves behind and penetrates her vagina from the rear. His fist continues to batter her genitals from the front and he crashes into her from behind as if he is a battering ram. Her neck is arching upwards, her mouth opening and suddenly she screams piercingly, over and over again. She shrieks and howls, she is so loud she is disturbing. Her body actually shakes and ricochets with the force of her climax, each contraction shooting her body forwards and then back again. And she doesn't stop, she continues jerking abruptly forwards until her screaming sounds quite worn out and she can hardly move. Which is just as well because her partner, who has been thrusting so hard that she has moved halfway across the mattress, judders his

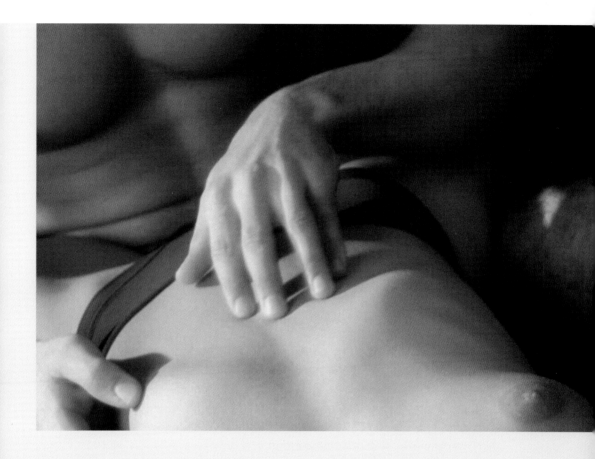

way to a climax, shouting 'Oh' at the top of his voice with every involuntary contraction of his ejaculation. A short while after they have collapsed in a heap, she crawls into his sheltering arm and looks up at him with enormous satisfaction. 'Mmm,' she says, licking her lips. 'Mmm,' He grins and closes his eyes.

Is this how you have sex? Can you let go like this couple? Or is your pattern quieter and softer? What do you think such rough sex might feel like? Could it be an option for you? If the answer is no, think about why not? Would you fear it? Would it turn you on at all? Or is the following visualization more recognizable?

The Fairy Fuck

A hotel room – the door opens and a petite dark-haired woman walks in, followed by a large older man. In close-up, you realize she is Japanese. The couple put down their suitcases and she experimentally sits on the bed. 'It's good,' she says, bouncing experimentally. 'Nice and soft.' 'Good,' he comments, 'I'll be able to sleep.' The couple unpacks. She puts on her white nightdress, he his pyjama bottoms. They climb into bed and just as he is about to put out the light, she stops him. 'Not yet, darling.' He looks grumpy but acquiesces. She leans over him and kisses him. He responds a little reluctantly. You can practically see him glancing at his watch. But he kisses her back. Emboldened, she kisses him again and this time he embraces her more deeply. He kisses her long and passionately, so passionately that her little body begins to squirm inside its white cotton. 'Take this off,' he urges and, seizing the garment, drags it over her head. Without it you realize what a perfect body this young woman has – but in miniature. Placed against her husband's larger frame she looks like a fairy. He carries on kissing her, and while doing so, hauls her little body up on top of his. He pushes her hand towards his pyjama bottoms. She fumbles for the cord, undoes it and then slides down his body to pull off the cotton trousers. His erection is standing up – he is very broad with a wide head to his penis. 'Come on, darling,' he fumbles impatiently between her legs, rubs her briefly with his forefinger, withdraws the forefinger and looks at it. It is glistening with moisture. 'Umm,' he says, and puts the finger his mouth. 'Um.' He flirts with her and she is shy, but pleased. She shows her arousal by squirming her rear even harder until he seizes her tiny bottom, covering the buttocks with his big hands and quite gently steers her down onto his large cock. Each gasps as the tiny cunt encloses the big erection. She sits astride him for a while, moving energetically up and down. You catch glimpses of this large penis poking up her as she waves her buttocks energetically in a kind of frenzied massage. 'Lie down on me, darling,' grunts the man. 'Give me a kiss.' She stretches over him and he kisses her passionately, then pushes her with his hands upwards and downwards so that she is rubbing full frontal across him. 'Don't stop,' she gasps. Her tiny frame suddenly stops, freezes then quite slowly jerks –1 –2 –3. She says not a word, but her mouth is wide open in a wordless cry. He is watching this with love. And when she is finished, he pulls her up, off his penis and kisses her with affection. 'Better now, darling?' he says jokingly, and she smiles slowly and

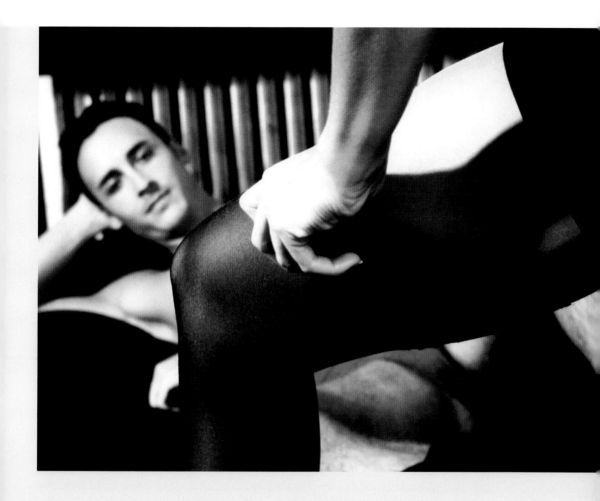

affectionately, too. 'Don't you want to come?' she asks. 'No, I don't think I do,' he replies. 'I'll save it for another occasion.'

What were you expecting to happen with this couple? Did you think that the older man might be going to take some kind of advantage of her? Who would you see as the protagonist here? And how did this sexual pattern feel to you? Was it different? Or was it familiar? Is this the kind of sex that you enjoy? Or would you like to enjoy it? Was it easier to relate to than the previous scene?

Cunnilingus

We see a tall, thin, young man with lanky long hair and a drooping moustache, walk hand-in-hand with his long-haired girlfriend into their bedroom. Outside the door we pause for a minute and listen in. He is coaxing her to take her clothes off. She says she doesn't want to, she's busy. 'Oh, come on, honey,' he pleads, 'Let's cuddle.' After a bit more grumbling, she reluctantly agrees. We go through the door as they lie down together. They kiss and cuddle but she's still not terribly interested. The young man looks at her knowingly, 'I know what you want.' Without saying anything more he slides down her body and parts her legs. We look at her genitals, nestling in a halo of dark, luxuriant curls. He raises his left arm so that his hand curves above her clitoris and with thumb and forefinger draws back the top of her pubic mound exposing the tiny glistening button that is her clitoris. She puts her hands on his head and her fingers wrap themselves in his hair. He lower his head to her crotch and pointing his tongue, pushes upward with it against her clitoris. 'Oh yes,' she says. Now she is interested. His head with his tongue projecting forward moves up and down, up and down, always running up and along the underside of her tiny clitoris. Which is not now so tiny. You can actually see it swell to twice its normal size. Now he pushes his tongue up first one side of the clitoris, then the other side. Then he twirls his tongue in tiny circles on the top of the clitoral head. She is breathing hard now, her left hand repeatedly rubbing around and around her left breast. He glances up and sees that her eyes are closed and that she is far off, away in her head. He goes back to the original licking up underneath the clitoris and over the head before retreating downward again. She loves this and curls her legs around his head, almost throttling him. He manfully keeps going as she begins to jerk her hips. 'More, please,' she gasps, 'More.' He obliges by ramming his head and tongue up and down even faster. If there were sexual stamina records this guy would be breaking them. Finally she gasps, 'I'm coming, I'm coming!' and then moans 'Oh,' 'Oh,' 'Oh,' in time to tiny jerks of her buttocks and hips. He gives signs he is about to stop. 'No,' she shrieks and pushes his head down, 'Keep going.' He laboriously carries on and she rewards him by quietly experiencing several more neat jerks of the buttocks. Finally he is allowed to halt and she draws him up so that his head is next to hers. You see that his face is hot and sweaty and that his mouth and lower part of his face covered with her juices. 'You're gorgeous, Roy,' she says, taking his head between her hands, kissing him square on

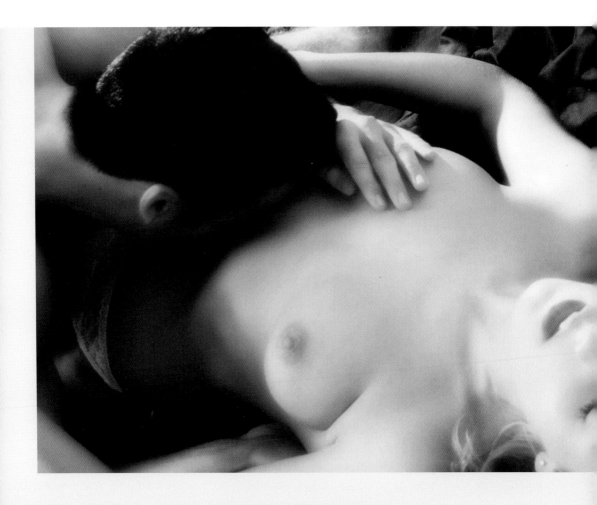

her own love lubes. Roy is almost too tired to notice, although at the end of this scene, he does go on to have missionary position sex with her for his own orgasm.

Is this how oral sex goes for you? Would you use other techniques that Roy omitted? How do you feel about the mess, the lubrication, the juxtaposition of genitals and lips? The idea of tasting the other person's interior juices? Have you ever tasted your own? If not, have a think about why not. Give it a go.

Fellatio

We zoom in on an older woman and a younger man. He is a lot younger, possibly 20 years younger. She is youthful-looking but middle-aged. They are walking naked into a living room. They are laughing, carrying glasses of wine and touching affectionately as they walk towards the sofa. She gestures towards it and laughingly pushes him to sit down. He knocks back a long draught of wine, then puts the glass down by the side of his seat. He's smiling wide and looking amused and appreciative of what is to come. He pats the side of the sofa inviting her next to him but she declines and sinks to her knees in front of him. Putting a hand on his thigh, she urges him to shuffle forward on his bottom so that his pelvis is half off the edge of the sofa with his genitals protruding towards her. Neither appears remotely embarrassed but look instead as if they anticipate a really fun time. Pushing open his legs so that they are wide, she lowers her mouth onto his flaccid penis. It is quite small at present and appears to fit rather well. She smiles with her mouth full, and holding the base with one hand, draws her mouth back from it. She also slides her other hand in underneath his testicles and on each up movement of her head, moves the hand up and away underneath the testicles. He reacts almost immediately to her skill and his penis telescopes before our eyes. A little more sucking and rubbing and his erection is so hard it already looks at bursting point. It has gone a deep purple and is straining. At one point she stops, takes her mouth away and looks at the tip. The entrance to the penis is gleaming and lubricated. She squeezes him slightly and beads of fluid appear in the tiny hole. 'Don't stop,' he groans and tries to move her head back down. Now she is sliding her head up and down to meet the hand gripping the base of the penis. She is pumping hard on him and sucking like a vacuum cleaner. Her hand slides up to meet her head coming down and the combined sucking, rubbing and swirling of opposite movements, vacuums him completely out of his mind so that he erupts into her mouth. As he ejaculates, she keeps still and concentrates on holding his come in her mouth. When his penis slowly deflates, she helps him out and then spits his come neatly onto a Kleenex. He is slumped against the back of the sofa, his head back, breathing hard but slowing down. She rests her head, tired from hard movement, against his naked thigh. His limp cock has fallen behind her and gleams with saliva and come. His hand raises slowly and pats her quietly on the shoulder. She nods her head silently. They don't need to talk. They are comfortable.

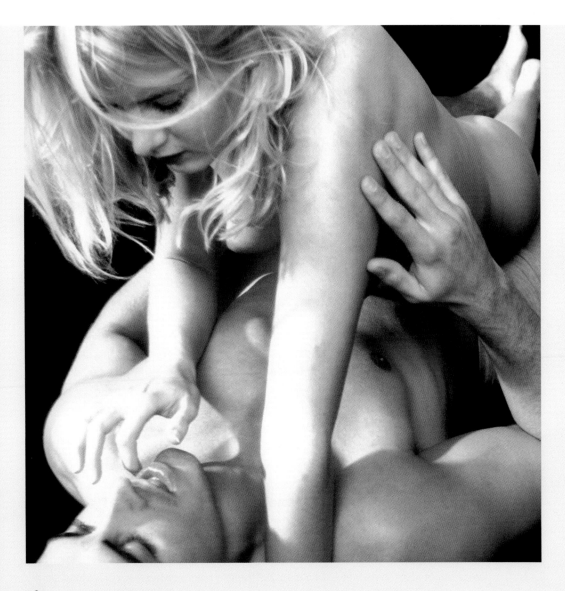

What are your thoughts here? Is this a usual picture of oral sex? How did you feel about the relationship between an older woman and a younger man? What thoughts/emotions went through your head? Was there anything that felt wrong about what you saw? Could you deal with giving or receiving fellatio?

Homosexuality

Two gay men are sprawled across a king-size bed looking at a magazine. They are in their 30s, sturdily built and one is a little taller than the other. The bigger guy has a shaven head while the other shows off a college boy hairstyle. They are naked and their buttocks gleam intensely white in contrast to the tan on the rest of their bodies. As your gaze travels along their backsides, you roll on up those pert white buns to take a look at their reading matter. They are looking at a gay magazine and in particular at the centrefold. Pictured on it is a young, handsome, well-groomed and exceedingly well-hung porno movie star. The guys are chuckling as they show the centrefold off to each other. They soon grow bored and move on to other spreads; one catches their attention and they stop flicking through the book. You sense that each is getting turned on by the picture, since their bodies go very still. The smaller man grins, then rubs the other guy's hand over his now enlarging cock. What is it that is such a turn-on? Peering over their shoulders you see a spread of photos, depicting a muscular black man sliding his muscular penis in between the buttocks of a smaller white man. The pictures portray the in-and-out of penile thrusting, and the last of the series, shows the black man head back, gripping the white guy around the waist and straining him against his body as he evidently comes.

'I like that,' says our big guy. 'Yeah,' agrees the younger guy and, turning towards his friend, kisses him passionately, long and full on the lips. 'It's a good one.' The couple kiss a great deal, on the mouth, on the neck and on the chest. As they do so, they rub and pull at each other's nipples until these stand up with small erections of their own. The big guy puts his head down and sucks on his friend's breast until his friend is gasping and squirming with sensation. The big guy has lost his erection though his friend's looks swollen enough for two. On seeing this, the friend drops to his knees and swiftly sucks and manipulates his mate's cock. The erection returns, unfolding like an inflatable. Now the big guy spits on his hand, rubs that hand across his friend's rear, and then, having sucked on his forefinger first, puts this finger, dropping spittle, into his friend's back passage. He slips and twists and winds his way, inch by inch, into the depths of his friend's resistant arse. 'Stop, wait,' are the gasped commands when the pressing finger gets too much. But it doesn't wait long to go on and soon that probing digit is stretching and widening his friend's rosebud rear. He is rimming, moving his finger round and round the immediate inside of the anus, conjuring up every shred of sensual feeling from a highly sensuous region. 'Oh, my God!' his friend is gasping, 'Oh, my God.' When he hears this, Big guy reckons his friend is ready to receive him, and buttering up his cock with gobs of saliva he carefully pushes his penis into his mate's now helpless backside. His mate is still lying on his back and raises his legs high while the big guy pushes in as if he were having hetero intercourse. As he presses deeper, his friend's eyes almost roll back in their sockets thanks to the deep sensation that is sending him almost out of his skull. Big guy's first withdrawal and then second thrust are tentative. Small guy has to get used to him. But his arse

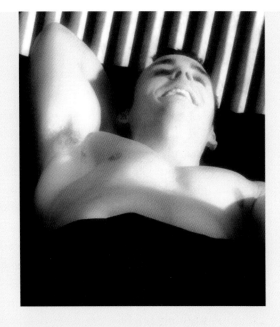

eases up and soon Big guy is thrusting, with Small guy's legs wrapped like snakes around his broad shoulders. It only takes about four deep thrusts for Small guy to go out of his skin with his climax. He wedges his hands somewhere in between the two of them and attempts to catch the ejaculate that is swamping his torso. Big guy looks down and likes what he sees, and shoving his head back, gives a last almighty heave and roars, bucking and jerking as he does so. After the sex has finished the two guys lie together a while. Big guy turns to his friend, gives him a peck on the cheek and says, 'That was great, honey,' and you can tell that he means it.

Does this feel like porn when you read it, or not? Is the experience utterly alien, or do you own up to feelings of fascination? In case you doubt that men can have sex like this, don't. They can and do. Could you ever imagine yourself doing this? Just because you can imagine it, does not mean you will ever do it. But many of us are actually bisexual, yet so well conditioned by the society we've grown up in that those other sexual feelings never get permission to come on out. Or is it the last kind of sex you have ever wanted to know about? Look hard at all your feelings. Where are you on the Kinsey scale of gender inclination? Gay, bisexual or straight?

Lesbianism

The first thing you hear are screams of laughter and the drumming of feet. Then more screams and giggles and 'Got you.' The sound of pouncing and tickling and someone screaming hysterically at the top of their voice. When you look round the door two women in their late 20s, one of average build, the other very skinny, are chasing each other round the room. They are fully clothed in tight cotton tops and loose-fitting trousers. The skinny woman with a mop of short curly hair stumbles on to the sofa, where she is mercilessly tickled by her friend. She is so helpless with laughter that soon she begs her friend to stop. 'If you don't stop,' she says, 'I'll wet myself. I can hardly control myself. Please, please,' she begs. 'Oh, I can see a little bit of wet,' her friend teases, pretending to look hard at her friend's crotch. 'You can't, can you?' her helpless partner, both frightened and unbelieving and still giggling weakly. 'Not really,' says her mate and takes pity by stopping her manic finger action. 'Oh, thank God,' Skinny sighs with relief. It's an effort to haul herself upright. She leans exhausted on her friend's shoulder for a couple of minutes and then nudges her mouth onto her friend's neck. She nuzzles into it, absent-mindedly kissing and softly biting it. Her tickling partner doesn't take a lot of notice to begin with but relaxes into the sensation, until she turns her head swiftly sideways, puts a hand under her friend's chin and draws Skinny into a huge kiss. Skinny melts like a jelly on a hot day until she is flopped right down into her friend's body. Her friend stops, appraises her, and smiles. It's the sort of smile that shows she is feeling very powerful with this friend whom she can reduce to a heap. Slowly and deliberately she leans forward and kisses Skinny hard and square on the lips. Then she bites, hard enough to make Skinny scream and leap back. 'Why did you do that?' 'Because you're good enough to eat,' says her friend. 'So I'm going to do just that.' And is back to chasing a hysterical Skinny halfway across the room. This time when she gets her friend in an armlock in a corner Skinny kisses and then bites right back. 'Bitch,' screams her friend but she's smiling. Holding Skinny's arms behind her back, she unties the drawstring on Skinny's loose-fitting cotton trousers and gets her friend to step out of them. Since Skinny is not wearing panties, you can see that on her almost skeletal pelvis there is a great bush of brilliant red pubic hair. Her friend looks at this admiringly. Meanwhile, the owner of the red pubes has fallen silent. 'You are gorgeous, you know,' says her lover and proceeds to take off her own cotton trousers. Leading her mate back to the sofa she sits her down then sits next to her. One arm around her shoulders she kisses Skinny a lot more until Skinny is squirming. 'Rub me, Matty,' pleads Skinny. Matty obliges. She puts her fingers into Skinny's flaming pubes and rubs backwards and forwards but very, very lightly as if she is just skimming her fingertip over the surface of Skinny's genitals. Skinny looks intent. Matty changes the up and down movement of her finger to circling with a fairy lightness on the tip of Skinny's clitoris and Skinny almost passes out with sensuality. She lies absolutely still, so still you wonder if she has fainted, but as Matty continues with the delicate finger work Skinny spreads her arms out wide, and her legs out wide and climaxes from the very heart of her body. You can see her contract in ripples that flood across her abdomen and out through her arms. And she cries with sounds that are wrenched from the back of her throat. Wordless, meaningless sounds that pierce the air in the room exactly as the climax appears to be piercing her body. Then, very, very lightly, she subsides and is quite silent. Her friend settles calmly down beside her. Within a minute, Skinny turns to Matty and puts both arms around her. 'I love you, Matty,' she says. 'I love you.'

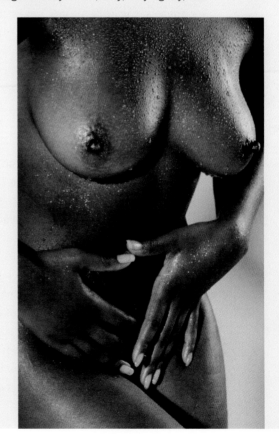

Did this feel more or less shocking than the two guys having sex? Was there anything unexpected in the scene you have just read about? Did anything feel wrong about this love-making between two women, or did it feel entirely natural to you? Did it turn you off, turn you on or leave you indifferent? How do you feel now? What do you think about the fact that one of the women has not climaxed?

A Threesome

There's a party. People are dancing, drinking, smoking and talking intently, trying to make themselves heard above the hubbub. We close in on one particular small group who are seated on a huge sofa at the back of the room where they are half-hidden by the sheer numbers packing the room. They aren't saying much these three, just smiling softly, drinking wine and watching the others. There are two good-looking dark-haired men in their late 30s, dressed in soft black T-shirts and black trousers. And a woman, aged around 40, wearing a halter top that leaves her back bare and a skirt down to the ground. When your eyes get used to the cigarette smoke, you notice that one of the men is caressing the woman's hand while the other is softly stroking her thigh underneath the folds of the material. What's more, the two guys are caressing each other's hands lying along the top of the sofa. No one is in a hurry. The woman puts down her wine glass and lies back. They stroke some more. She closes her eyes and basks in their touch. She virtually purrs. One man leans his head forward and kisses her on the mouth. She responds with surprising strength considering the lack of any other move of her own. Across her head the two guys meet eyes. One gestures and points upwards. 'Upstairs,' he suggests. The other nods faintly, and with his arms firmly around the woman, says, 'Let's go, Hilda.' She smiles faintly, nods and gathers up her bag. The three cross the crowded room, smile at acquaintances and walk upstairs to the comparative peace and quiet of low lighting and empty rooms. In the big dark bedroom the door is locked and the three move towards the bed. One man clasps her from behind and she lies back in his protective arms. The other stands in front of her and clasps both the woman and the man in his embrace. He stands in front of her, but his arms caress his male friend. She puts her arms around his neck and kisses him. Long kisses later, the two men take off their trousers. But when she attempts to disrobe from her evening skirt, one of them stops her. 'No,' he says, 'Leave it on.' But he does help her step out of her panties. While one man continues to kiss and fondle her through her clothes, the other lifts up her skirt and caresses her buttocks. Leaning forwards he curves his arm around underneath the skirt and you can tell from the movement in the material that he is slowly stroking her vagina in long, relaxed strokes. Occasionally you get glimpses of her long legs as the skirt rises and falls. She is finding it harder and harder to remain standing up right. She staggers a little and the man kissing now holds her steady. She is moan-

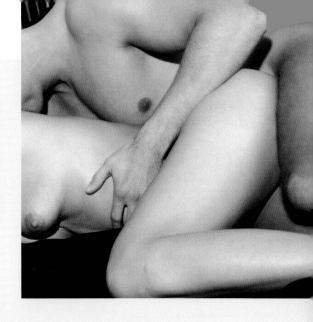

ing and softly sighing, and getting more turned on by the minute. Her moans turn to distinct cries and the cries get more and more rapid and urgently loud. The men are telling her how attractive she is, and the more they talk about how hard they desire her the more carried away she becomes. She really can hardly stand now so the front man sits on the floor and helps her down with him. He slips off his boxers and lying flat, gently pulls her on top of him. With a billowing of her skirt over his abdomen she settles down slowly, her cunt closing down on his penis.

The man at the back of her is helping her get into place. He is holding her hips and as he does so looks at the other male who smiles back. Now the man at the rear lifts up the skirt and kneeling over her legs, slowly drives his penis into her rear. He manages this without any great difficulty. You get the sense that she has done this many times before. But no matter how many times, the sensation of being so filled, in both front and back passages really does it for this woman. She stays quite still while the rear guy drives into her and comes quickly to his orgasm. As he shouts his climax the other guy who has been watching is visibly moved. As soon as the rear guy has withdrawn he encourages her to move rapidly on top of him so that she can whip him into his own climax. She does this while now fingering herself so that she can get an orgasm of her own. He comes very quickly indeed and the man underneath, seeing her climax, seizes her by the hips and ejaculates deep into her. Both are crying out as they come. When it's over, the rear guy helps her wipe herself down with a tissue and then helps his male friend. For a short time the three lie relaxed together on the floor until one of them says, 'We should get back to the party.'

Is this how you imagined a threesome? If it's not, how does your version differ? Is this something you would like to experience or are you happy to leave it to others? Is there anything about this scene you are uncomfortable with? What role do you think the woman is playing? What do you think she means to the two men? And what does she get out of this?

Senior Sex

A much older couple are drinking tea and smoking a cigarette. They are naked. You would guess that she is around 60 and he is probably 70. Their bodies are just the bodies of older people, wrinkled but tanned. Their faces, however, light up when they smile making both look very attractive. They also look very affectionate towards each other. They pat each other's hand often, kiss, cuddle and joke together. Ultimately she gets up and pulls him up after her. They are both grinning as they walk into the bedroom. This older couple spends a good half-hour caressing, giving each other a lot of hand manipulation; she particularly gives him a lot of oral sex before his erection gets really hard. And when he comes before she does, he continues afterwards to bring her to orgasm with his hand. They seem open and natural and comfortable with their bodies. They clearly have a great time together and enjoy each other a lot. When they finish, you go away thinking what a great marriage this couple has. You can almost feel the tangible affection that they express towards each other through their sex. So it comes as quite a surprise afterwards when you hear that they are not married, they are just very good old friends.

JOIN THE GROWN-UPS

It is this less judgemental attitude towards sex that allows you to look at sexual situations and sexual problems with greater ease than you have managed before. One of the ultimate tests is when you can manage to talk to your parents about sex. I am not suggesting you go into explicit details you know will shock and offend them. They haven't just read the visualization programme. But you are all grown-ups now. You should be able to feel comfortable enough to hold some conversation about sex.

Does it shock you that a so-much older man and woman could have such enjoyable sex without being in a committed relationship? How do you think that they coped with not having perfect bodies? It's one thing for a long-term partner to be used to the shape of your body – you get to feel comfortable with him/her. But a new partner? What will they think about our lumps and bumps? And yet this couple seemed absolutely fine together. What does it take to behave in this way?

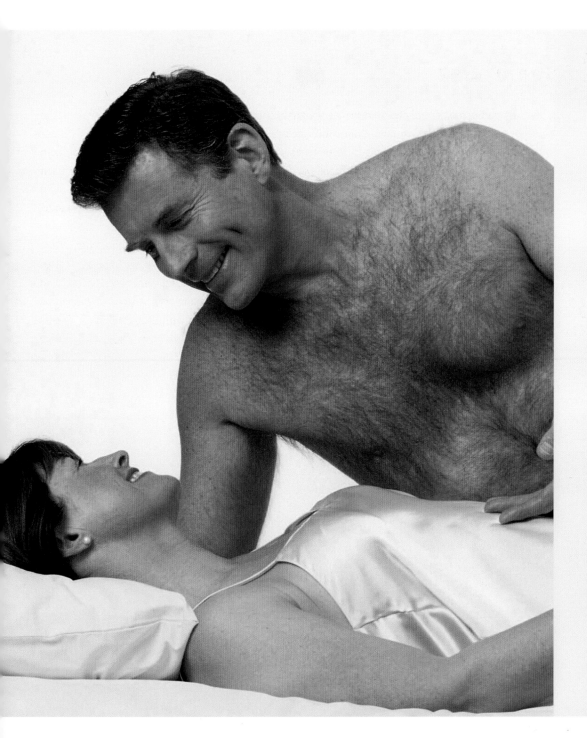

What You've Learned

You have now read through a short collection of visualizations. Ideally there should be many more, in fact an entire volume full. Here, alas, we don't have the space. But I hope you begin to get an idea of what I'm aiming at. You have probably read the visualizations to yourself, in private. Do you notice any difference in the way you were feeling about the sexual activities described at the end of the series compared to the feelings that you experienced at the beginning? Were you feeling less turned on as you continued with your reading? And more able to look at what was going on dispassionately?

If you don't notice much change in your reactions this may be because I can only present a short selection here and I would suggest you go back to the beginning and read through this again. After this, I would then suggest that if you haven't already done so you read through the visualizations once more only this time with other people – that you all read and then discuss these as a group. In between each subject, stop and discuss what you've just imagined and voice your feelings – the thoughts, fears, hopes that the descriptions evoke.

It is when you can talk about these taboo subjects openly with no embarrassment or shame, that you know your attitudes to sex are changing.

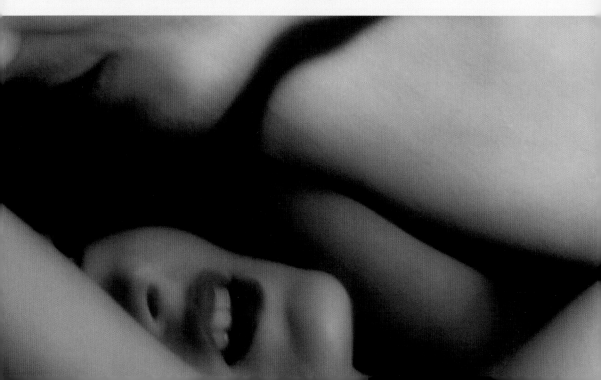

Of course, you do need to temper your discussion to what other people may be able to accept. But my own experience of this is that it is quite possible to talk explicitly about sex, without using crude words or expressions in a way that can be acceptable. I certainly know that when you feel comfortable with sex, other people settle down and start to feel comfortable too.

And just so that you don't think I've included the visualizations as unadulterated porn, here is the theory behind them. It is only by becoming familiar with sexual behaviours that you can get used to them. And it is only by getting used to these that the heat, the sting, goes out of such activities. Instead of seeing them as shameful, they become just sexual behaviour. The guilt-laden judgements that you have unconsciously brought to them eases away. So my reason for writing the visualizations is to give you an inkling, in print, between these pages, of what the SAR programme does with much greater efficiency and immediacy through film.

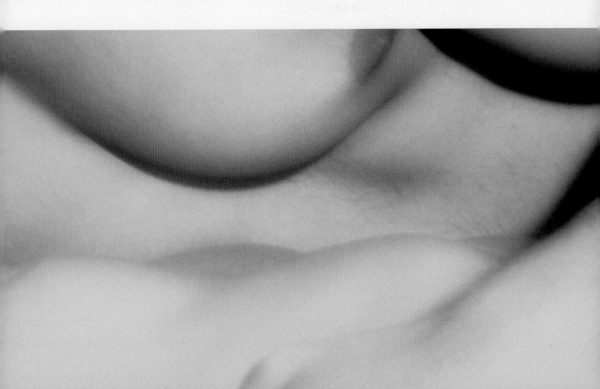

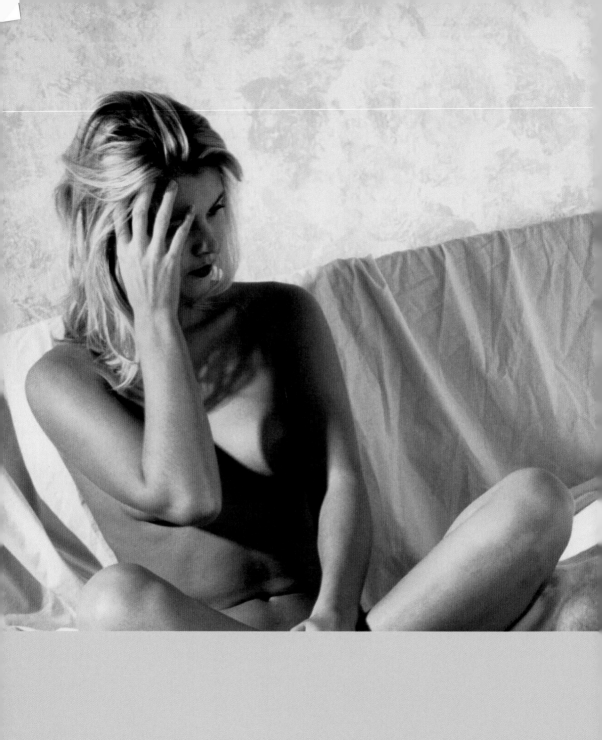

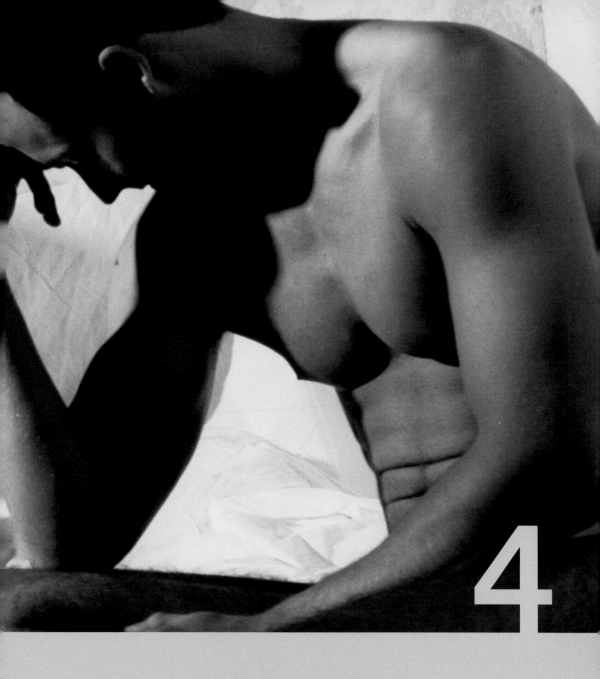

4

When Sex Goes Wrong

Who is in Control of Your Body?

Have you ever dreamed of dressing your partner up in a black mask, fixing straps between his or her buttocks and tying them to the bedpost before fucking the life out of him or her? Come on – admit it. You can do so here because no one will ever know. But even if you don't admit it, I wouldn't mind betting that the reality is that you have never dared to actually do this. Thinking is one thing – carrying it out quite another. So what do you suppose is stopping you?

The answer might be common sense. You are absolutely certain that your partner would run a mile the minute you whipped out the cat o' nine tails. And it's a good answer. But suppose you don't know this? Suppose you only think this because you believe that only abnormal people would do such outrageous things and you would rather die than have anyone think you were so outrageous? Who or what exactly is preventing you now?

Let's go further. Let's suppose your partner secretly felt the same and was only waiting for you to make the suggestion? There you are, two people who might be enjoying an exceptional sexual intimacy and yet are completely blocked. You would hurt no third party if you followed your real desire but something inside is stopping you. That something is the force of what you believe to be public opinion.

Constrained, Controlled and Prescribed Sex

Public opinion may turn out to be a powerful meme. It can certainly dictate any number of opposite beliefs depending on what part of the world you live in. If you believed that everyone in your country went to an S and M club every Saturday night, then the odds are you'd be there too. Or look at it another way. You have no trouble with having sex in the missionary position – everyone knows that this is the ordained Western method of having sex. So imagine visiting a society where everyone found the missionary position entirely shocking yet you were the only one to use it? Wouldn't the censure of everyone around seem ridiculous? Yet as you think about it a little more, mightn't you begin to feel that perhaps missionary sex could be depraved and wrong in certain circumstances?

We are a species who so much wants to feel ourselves in line
that we sometimes go along with ideas we know deep down
are nonsense.

However, I now want to complicate the issue. So far I've been arguing about the dramatic decisions we may wrestle with in our sex lives. But suppose our predilections are the opposite. Suppose, in fact, that sex isn't all that interesting to us. Haven't there been times when you really wished you didn't have to perform that night and aren't there other times when you prefer to curl up with a good book and a box of chocolates or spend time on your computer playing games?

Some people don't feel sex is their priority. They are perfectly comfortable with a life that includes little of it. Yet other people find it hard to let them be. These more laidback, less sexually driven individuals either get pressured into finding a sex partner or are made to feel they are seriously lacking if they don't. Men foolish enough to reveal they have a short penis or a low sex drive become the butt of jokes, the subject of innuendo. Colleagues make fun of them behind their backs. Women who rarely experience orgasm are not infrequently made to feel as if something is seriously wrong with them. And these criticisms are often made when the women themselves are not terribly bothered about their quieter sex lives. They are actually penalized for being well-adjusted.

Somewhere along the line the idea has seeped through that men and women who are not overly sexual are inadequate. But the truth is that these are normal people. They are at one end of the normal human spectrum of sexuality. This doesn't stop others dictating what choices should be made for them. And the minute anyone starts feeling he or she ought to be performing better it is because he or she is being subjected to just as powerful a controlling constraint as those men and women who don't dare to snap on the handcuffs.

GENITAL SIZE

There are other spectrums of sexuality, too. Penis size ranges from the microphallus to the 30-cm/12-inch ruler. Different races are found to have different penis shapes and lengths. As long as they are all in working order who is to say anything is wrong with any of them. Clitoral size ranges, too. The average clitoris is 3.75 cm/1½ in long, and labia vary greatly in size and shape.

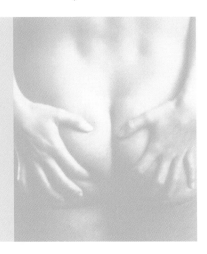

CASE HISTORY

Sheila and Tom were referred for sex therapy because Tom complained Sheila didn't ever want sex and Sheila complained their sex life didn't work for her. On questioning, it turned out that the couple regularly had intercourse and Sheila regularly enjoyed orgasm. Their sex life did work. What then was wrong? Tom explained that Sheila never made the moves in bed, never initiated sex. He complained about this several times. Sheila, on the other hand, revealed that although she could be physically aroused, Tom didn't really turn her on emotionally. Tom moaned and whined about what a bad wife she was because she didn't want sex all the time – as he did. He sounded like a demanding little boy.

When I analysed their complaints, the problem boiled down to his ideas about the kind of sexuality a good wife provides for her man. As a favoured younger child, he had literally been spoon-fed. He had had everything done for him by his mother. Now he expected his wife to do the same. His meme was that he believed a good wife derived her pleasure from her man's pleasure. If he felt erotic so, too, did she. And if he needed a lot of reassurance in the shape of sexuality, well then, naturally, she would want to give it all the time, wouldn't she?

I encouraged this couple to concentrate on and build up the areas that functioned well. Tom worked on not asking for sex so often and also became better at giving Sheila climaxes. Sheila, in turn, accepted that Tom was an anxious man who needed a lot of reassurance. She made a point of giving him more reassurance in general so that eventually he didn't need so much sexual reassurance because he finally felt she cared about him.

Sexual Spectrums

Every jot of research into the patterns of human sexuality shows that men and women experience extraordinarily diverse patterns of sexuality. Alfred Kinsey, who did major research in the late 1940s and early 1950s, deduced, after taking thousands of case histories, that there is a spectrum of human sexuality just as there is of colour or health or intelligence. It is as human to want to play extreme sex games as it is also human to only want sex twice a year. Yet even while you read this, I bet that many of you will almost immediately reject the thought as nonsense. That is how deep our beliefs are entrenched.

Another of Kinsey's spectrums measured gender orientation. He saw normal human sexuality running from heterosexuality on one side of the spectrum through bisexuality in the middle, right across to homosexuality on the spectrum's opposite side.

Other surveys have shown that, as far as acts of sex are concerned, individuals ranged between none per year right through to five acts per day, every day. These latter were not all acts of intercourse but included masturbation and were relevant to a younger rather than an older age range with a few notable exceptions. It might be true to say that no act of sex at all, ever, is abnormal, except those that harm someone else.

Since we are a race that must perpetuate ourselves through sex, the only real perversity might be to never have sex at all.

But, of course, there is an evolutionary reason for that, too. Unmarried uncles and aunts are extremely valuable in an evolutionary sense because they could be assisting family genes to grow strong, even though they have no children of their own.

If you have a lower sex drive, and you marry someone else with a lower sex drive, then there is no problem. You match each other perfectly. The real difficulties arise if you:

- Get together with a partner who does not perfectly match you;
- Find a partner who is too inhibited to say what is really on his/her mind;
- Feel so pressurized that your sexual performance just wilts.

Looked at from the starting point of ideas, you are being affected by notions or beliefs in all these situations. It is the ideas you possess about sexuality that trouble you – not the actual sexual performance.

If we want to examine what is going wrong in our sex lives, we need to begin with the entire concept of a sexual belief system. If you can identify your own or your partner's sex-

COMMON SEX **myths**

Below are a few of the memes that I have come across during 20 years of sex counselling. They begin with "If I...

- Do anything he/she wants in bed he/she will stay faithful;
- Refuse to do something he/she wants in bed, then he/she definitely will leave me;
- Cannot rise to the occasion every time, I am not a real man;
- Cannot climax at the same time as my partner, I am not doing sex properly;
- Ejaculate before 20 minutes of thrusting, I am a poor lover;
- Cannot swallow semen during oral sex, my man will think me a poor lover;
- Have a succession of one-night stands, I can prove I am independent;
- Don't constantly introduce novelty to the sex act, I will lose my partner's interest;
- Constantly initiate new sexual ideas, my partner will think I'm a slut;
- Don't constantly initiate new sexual ideas, my partner will believe me unmanly.

ual beliefs, you get an inkling of the memes that are driving them – and, at second-hand, the memes that are therefore also driving you, whether or not you approve of them. How do we avoid falling into these traps? Is it even possible to do so? The realistic answer is that we all grow up in specific families and cultures. We can't help absorbing ideas from that culture. We do so from the very start of life as tiny children. So the first step is to realize that to make adult life work sometimes we need to change our ideas and move on. We can only do that provided we know what those ideas consist of. To do that a little self-analysis is called for. Take a look at my sexual memes test in Chapter Two, and when you have identified some of the sexual ideas that have influenced you during your upbringing, move on to the next section.

Know Your Own Sexual Beliefs

Read through the lists of options on pages 90–91 and mark out those that apply to your background and upbringing. There is no one right answer to these choices. You may want to mark out more than one choice because both beliefs may be operating side by side. By combining your ticked choices, you can get a handle on what your family taught you about sex without your even knowing it. I hope your family ethos becomes clearer after you have worked your way through these.

If you have identified beliefs picked up from your friends (see pages 92–93), take a further look at them and ask yourself in the light of today, are these actually practical in your present life? Do they have real meaning or are they based on superstition?

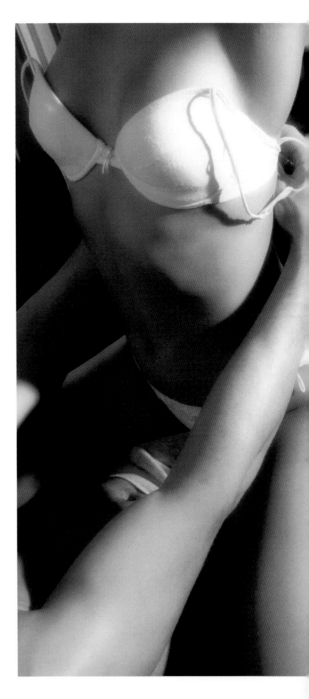

In My Family They Believe:

☐ Men are initiators and women passive.
☐ Women are initiators and men are passive.
☐ Both sexes take equal responsibility for initiating sexual activity.

☐ Men have much stronger sex drive than women.
☐ Women have much stronger sex drive than men.
☐ Men and women's sex drives are very similar.

☐ Men mainly want sex and women mainly want love.
☐ Men and women want sex and love in equal measure.
☐ Men mainly want love and women mainly want sex.

☐ Men are expected to have several sex relationships including extra-marital ones but women are expected to have few and to stay faithful.
☐ Women are expected to have several sex relationships including extra-marital ones but men are expected to have few and to stay faithful.
☐ Men are expected to always stay sexually faithful once married, as are women.
☐ Both sexes are likely to have other sexual partners during marriage.

☐ Infidelity is a hurdle to be got over.
☐ Infidelity is grounds for immediate separation.
☐ Infidelity is painful but can be dealt with provided it only happens once.

☐ Women are expected to nurture men sexually but not to expect much sexual nurturing themselves.
☐ Men are expected to take care of the woman's sexual needs regardless of their own.
☐ Men and women should take equal responsibility for each other's sexual needs.
☐ Men and women should take responsibility for their own sexual needs and expect the other to do so too.

☐ Sex is mainly a physical outlet.
☐ Sex is a comfort in times of anxiety.
☐ Sex is an expression of love.
☐ Sex is a method of domination.
☐ Sex is mainly necessary for good health.
☐ Sex is strictly for procreation.
☐ Sex is an ecstatic, almost religious experience.
☐ Sex is fun.

☐ Good sex should be taken for granted.
☐ Good sex needs constant care and work put into it.
☐ Good sex can only be spontaneous.

☐ If you love each other, everything will come right.
☐ If something goes wrong sexually, you should keep this private.
☐ If something goes wrong sexually, you should talk about it together.
☐ If something goes wrong, you should talk about it with a therapist.

☐ It is wrong to tell children about sex.
☐ It is wrong not to tell children about sex.
☐ You should wait until a child reaches puberty before telling them about sex.

☐ Nice people do not talk about sex openly.
☐ Nice people talk about sex as freely as they do about food.
☐ Nice people should pick their moments to discuss sexuality.
☐ Nice people do not talk about sex to their parents.
☐ Nice people do not talk about sex to their children.

From My Friends I Learned (Peers Beliefs):

☐ You should have as much sex as possible as soon as possible.
☐ You should save yourself until marriage.
☐ You should wait for the right person (i.e. until you fall in love and only then have sex).

☐ It is normal for boys to go through a homosexual phase.
☐ It is normal for girls to go through a lesbian phase.
☐ It is normal for girls and boys to pass through homosexual phases on the way to heterosexuality.
☐ It is normal for some boys and girls to remain either homo- or bisexual.
☐ It is abnormal for boys and girls to remain either homo- or bisexual.
☐ It is abnormal for girls and boys to go through any phase other than that of developing heterosexuality.

☐ It is normal to masturbate.
☐ It is abnormal to masturbate.
☐ Masturbation is OK provided it is seen as a phase to a more mature sexuality.
☐ Masturbation is not OK if you are in a committed relationship.
☐ Masturbation is great under any circumstances.

☐ It is fun to look at pornography.
☐ It is disgusting to look at pornography.
☐ It's OK to look at pornography provided you do it with your committed partner.
☐ Pornography is not OK in a committed relationship.
☐ It is the individual's choice about whether or not they want to look at pornography and as such should not adversely affect a committed partner.

☐ It is wrong to have sex anywhere other than in private.
☐ It is fine to have sex at parties.
☐ It is OK, in certain circumstances, to have sex in the same room as another couple.

☐ It is fine to take part in different types of sex provided you do so only with other like-minded people.

☐ It is healthy to enjoy sex in a threesome.

☐ It is normal to go through a phase of swinging.

☐ You will go to hell if you ever have sex with anyone other than your marital partner.

☐ It is OK for other people to experience these alternative sexual activities but it is not for you.

☐ It is fine to enjoy fetish sex either by yourself or with another provided you don't harm anyone.

☐ It is reasonable to ask a partner to join you in a fetish activity.

☐ It is unreasonable to pressurize a partner into fetish sex against his/her will.

☐ An interest in fetish sex is the sign of a sick mind.

☐ An interest in fetish sex is the mark of a progressive intelligence.

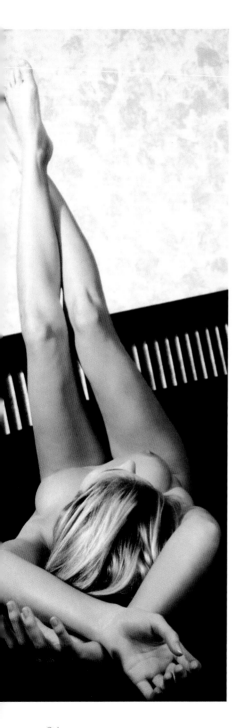

Fact or Fallacy?

Read through the following list and see if you can identify any myths that you believe to be true. Then have a look at what is, in fact, the truth.

FEMALE SEX **the myths**

Women:

- Must be passive for men to like and respect them;
- Should show no former knowledge of sexuality because that would make them appear 'bad';
- Should not ask for what they want in bed because that might make them sound demanding;
- Should wait for a man to express sexual interest before expressing any of their own;
- Find it hard to experience orgasm;
- Should possess perfect bodies to attract a man;
- Are nobody if they don't have a man;
- Should always please their men;
- Should fake orgasm if they can't actually experience one.

FEMALE SEX **the facts**

- Men usually love it when women take the sexual initiative.
- Men enjoy their woman delighting them with some choice sex practise.
- Women possess ordinary healthy sexual appetites just the same as men and are just as entitled to make their own sexual experiments.
- Women are responsible for their own sexuality.
- Women need to know their own sexual response so that they can bring this information into a relationship and lift some of the pressure off men. Although around 30 per cent of women only experience orgasm during intercourse alone, over 80 percent of women experience orgasm regularly through masturbation. Female orgasm usually requires specific clitoral stimulation that intercourse alone often does not provide due to poor fit between male and female sexual anatomy. The majority of women can and do experience orgasm during intercourse provided they are stimulated by hand prior to intercourse and/or during intercourse.
- Women are as attractive as they think they are. Proof of this is in the numbers of fat, thin and elderly women who manage to have terrific sex lives.
- Women in this day and age are finding more identity from work and less identity from marriage.
- It is good to please your lover but it is not always possible.
- The woman who fakes an orgasm, does her love life a disservice in the long-term because she is training her lover to do sex the wrong way.

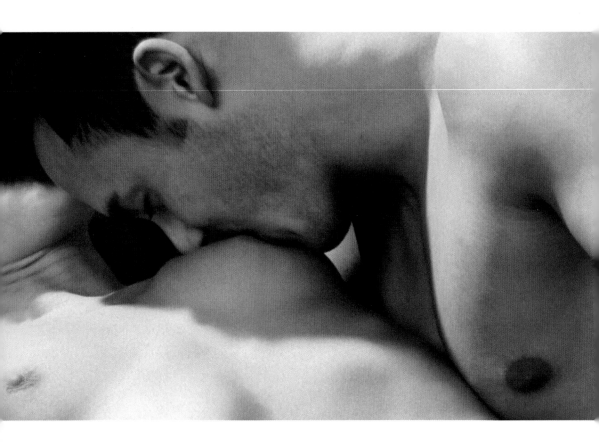

MALE SEX **the myths**

Men must:

- Be ever ready for sex;
- Be responsible for the woman's pleasure;
- Be hung like a bull to be sexually attractive;
- Always initiate, never be passive;
- Have dozens of sexual experiences;
- Always know what they are doing;
- Be in control.

MALE SEX **the facts**

- Men are entitled to their sexual moods just as women are, men cannot usually be sexually aroused unless there is someone or something specific that is attractive.
- Women need to be responsible for their own pleasure – not men, although it helps if men know what they are doing!
- Penis size is irrelevant, because it is what men do with their hands, mouth and entire body that counts to women. In a survey of what women find attractive in men, the greatest majority of men said they believed it was penis size that mattered most to women. Penis size, however, came virtually bottom of the list for women. Instead, they opted for buttocks as a source of visual turn-on.
- According to women, some of the sexiest men are those who feel sure enough about themselves to lie back and let the woman take charge.
- Too much sexual experience can be both daunting and anxiety-inducing for some women who fear they will a) not measure up against an array of other sexual relationships and b) are fearful of contacting the AIDS virus.
- Spontaneity in sex is much prized. A partner who is always in control leaves little room for spontaneity.

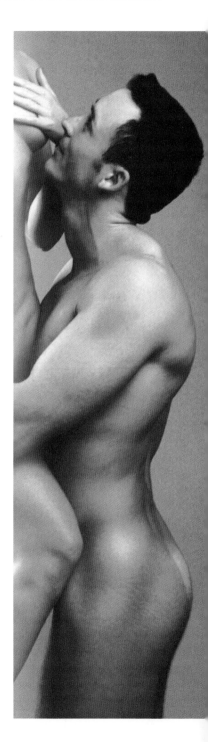

MASTURBATION **the myths**

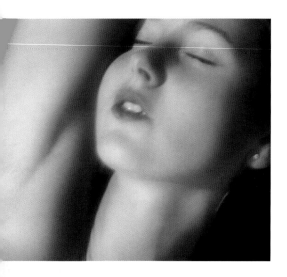

Everyone knows that masturbation:

- Can make you blind;
- Can make you ill or sap your energy;
- Can prevent you from being creative;
- Is only practised by sad, lonely people;
- Will make you so addicted you are unable to enjoy normal intercourse;
- Is a sign of nymphomania.

MASTURBATION **the facts**

- Masturbation causes no physical harm at all unless it is done so roughly that you actually wound yourself.
- It is a healthy, natural activity that far from preventing creativity or sapping energy probably relaxes the mind and body giving you better physical conditions with which to work or play.
- Masturbation actually provides the opportunity to explore and get familiar with your personal sexual response, and once you have managed this, it then allows you to take this knowledge into any subsequent relationship, thereby ensuring that the relationship has a greater likelihood of sexual success. It is, in this way, excellent training and rehearsal for a 'real' sexual relationship.
- Masturbation provides comfort and release for those without partners.
- Masturbation is not addictive.
- Although it is not a sign of nymphomania, masturbation may indicate a high sex drive.
- Masturbation can be a fulfilling ecstatic experience in its own right.

FANTASY **the myths**

A reliance on sexual fantasy is a sign of:

- Inadequacy; an inability to hold yourself in the here and now;
- Mental infidelity;
- An inability to experience pure sexual feeling for a partner;
- A sick mind.

FANTASY **the truths**

The ability to fantasize sexually is:

- Possibly the mark of a high testoterone count (for both males and females);
- Indicative of a creative imagination;
- Cannot be policed because the imagination is beyond conscious control;
- Probably a safeguard set up by the imagination to preserve long-term relationships when sex becomes repetitive;
- Possibly a safeguard for bottled-up feelings and desires that would not be socially acceptable.

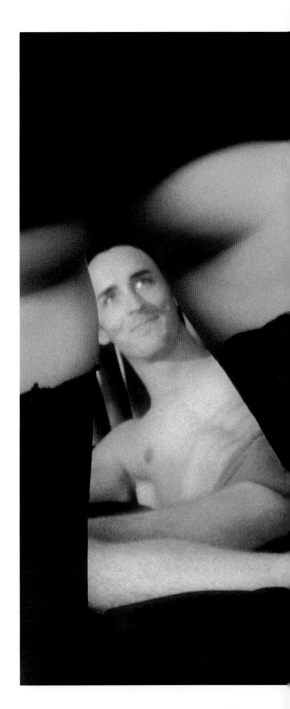

ORGASM **the myths**

What we know about orgasm is that:

- It must be experienced simultaneously;
- If you don't experience orgasm, you are inadequate;
- If you don't provide your partner with an orgasm, you are inadequate;
- A clitoral orgasm is inferior to a vaginal one;
- Women do not experience a proper orgasm since they do not ejaculate;
- Women cannot experience orgasm without foreplay;
- You must have an orgasm;
- The right way to have an orgasm is in the missionary position;
- A woman's genitals are ugly and so is her movement during orgasm;
- Orgasm means loss of control.

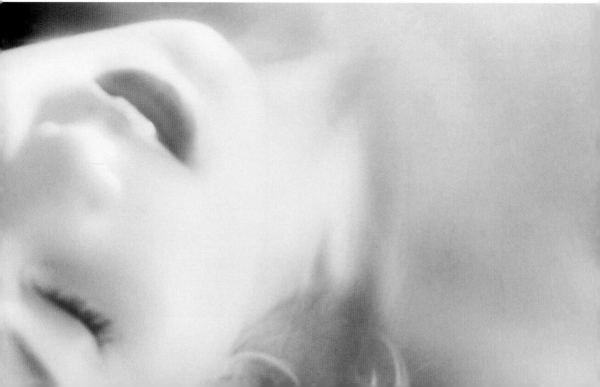

ORGASM **the facts**

- Orgasm can be experienced in any way, be it separately or simultaneously. Many people say that having to time an orgasm, so that it exactly coincides with that of a partner, often detracts from the full orgasmic sensation.
- There are many reasons for not experiencing orgasm and none of them have any bearing on an individual's self-worth.
- Each of us is responsible for our own orgasm. This means that if your partner does not experience one, it is up to him/her to improve things. Of course, it would be great to help, but in the end, his/her climax is his/her responsibility.
- There are many ways of experiencing climax, not just clitoral or vaginal and no one way is any better or any worse than another.
- Ejaculation is an old-fashioned definition of orgasm, especially since certain men climax without ejaculation and certain women with a very active G-spot appear to have an ejaculation.
- Some women can climax by thought (i.e. fantasy alone). Some women can climax by intercourse alone. Others can climax the minute a partner penetrates them.
- If orgasm becomes a must, the performance pressure this involves works against you. There should be no compulsion on anyone to have an orgasm. Sometimes we just don't feel like it.
- There is no 'right' way in which to have an orgasm. Any way is the 'right' way.
- Aesthetic taste is entirely personal. What is ugly to one individual is beautiful to another, and vice versa.
- In one sense, orgasm does mean a loss of control in that, at the moment of orgasm, we temporarily clock out to a different level of brain activity. But we never lose the ability to wrest ourselves straight back to earth if necessary as witnessed in the case of young mothers with crying babies.

A New Source of Sexual Love Patterns

Heterosexuals are usually so busy feeling superior they assume they are unlikely to learn from other groups of humans – and the last thing they would do is take a few tips from animals. That thought is literally abhorrent. Which is a pity, because men and women could learn something if they dared to let go of the insecurities on which their prejudices are founded.

Homosexual Love-Making

The US sex researchers Masters and Johnson, found during their research work on homosexual couples that homosexual and lesbian patterns of love making differed quite a bit from those of heterosexuals. When they launched their book, *Homosexuality in Perspective*, one of the publicity points much featured in the media was that the great sexologists considered heterosexual men and women could learn from homosexual love-making patterns. Homosexuals, it emerged, spent far more time on foreplay, exhibited more tenderness, and were happy to reach climax in many ways other than intercourse. Some couples would spend literally hours stroking each other's skin and building up sexual excitement with the thought of finishing the session (i.e. as in climax), far from their minds. Love-making was a whole-body experience and orgasm just one finalizing part of it.

Tips to follow:
- Make love without orgasm;
- Spend a two-hour period on massage alone;
- Practise stroking only certain limbs but stroke them often;
- Think of the whole body;
- Forget the genitals – these will manage to take care of themselves in the fullness of time;
- Curb impatience – this simply indicates that your mind is somewhere else and that you probably shouldn't be love-making at all right now.

As For The Animals...

In Bruce Bagemihl's fascinating book, *Animal Diversity*, the author documents the fact that, contrary to accepted belief, almost all animals exhibit homosexual behaviour. Much of this homosexual behaviour is specifically genitally oriented but not all. In the case of male giraffes, for example, Bagemihl poetically describes the twining and intertwining of those long graceful necks, snaking and undulating around each other's skin. What he describes, even though it may lead to sexual behaviour, is a type of sensuality. Since giraffes cannot be said to possess a higher consciousness, it could reasonably be argued that these animals are innocents. What happens innocently is not wrong. Human sensuality is not wrong either. When a little child unconsciously strokes his or her parent's arm, enjoying the pure sensation of the stroke, this is innocence. Our great sadness is that thanks to the layers of civilization, heaped on us by our 'intelligence', we lose this direct ability to communicate by sensual touch.

Touch more As 'grown-ups' we can't turn back the clock. We can't lose that conscious knowledge of what is considered sexually right or wrong. But we can try to set aside some prejudices and allow ourselves to be physically warmer, stroking dear friends of either sex. Men and women adore being touched. They react to caresses with feelings of powerful friendship. And just because you go out and hug a friend, this does not immediately mean that the friend receives 'the wrong idea'. Any idea that springs into his or her head will be partially dictated by your own attitude. If your attitude is that touch is a great way of conveying friendship but that is all, then that will come across. And if your friend resists this boundary, explain your philosophy. In the 1970s there was a great touchy feely movement emanating from California. Give a Friend a Hug Day was seriously celebrated. The most unlikely individuals found themselves in warm embraces. College professors, businessmen and politicians all managed it. And for just a few seconds, they enjoyed this rare contact.

So the message from the animals is to keep cuddling. The sensuality of cuddling does not have to be sexual. But it can feed all kinds of other emotional needs. You and your mates are likely to feel a lot better after a non-sexual cuddle. So risk trying it out. And watch what happens. If nothing else, life feels more satisfactory.

Getting Stuck in Sex Patterns in a Long-term Relationship

There is a lot of space given to research showing that men respond to novelty which is, of course, impossible in a well-established routine. In addition, men often experience a mid-life crisis during their forties when they suddenly pack in the old wife and take up with a newer, younger one. In contrast, there is also evidence that suggests that it is normal to settle on a continuing sex pattern. But there is absolutely no evidence to show that suddenly dressing up in black underwear and a mask makes the slightest difference to saving a marriage. If a marriage is going to continue, it is as likely to do so still using the same sex routine as not.

There might, however, be good reason for looking at the emotion underlying the marriage. Clair Hawes, a clinical psychologist from Vancouver, suggests improving the quality of a long-term relationship by concentrating on the small things that give it meaning. She suggests taking a look at some key areas around sexual intercourse, which you might be able to strengthen and improve.

These are:

- Sensitivity to each other's mood during intercourse;
- Carving out private time for intimacy;
- Deliberately giving each other's bodies more loving stimulation;
- Making a point of giving much greater stimulation to the genitals on the grounds that aging can mean diminished sexual sensation;
- Deliberately putting yourself in the way of sexual stimulation, such as sexy books or films which you can watch from your bed;
- Making love occasionally at times other than the usual ones;
- Taking a lot more holidays together. The break from routine can be stimulating.

MY SUGGESTION FOR LONG-TERM GOOD SEX

Appreciate the routine that has worked so well for you over the years and trust it. It is your routine. It works for you. If your relationship really is under threat, the dangers will be focussed on issues other than sex. Have faith in your idea of good sex. But don't be afraid to talk about the feelings underneath it.

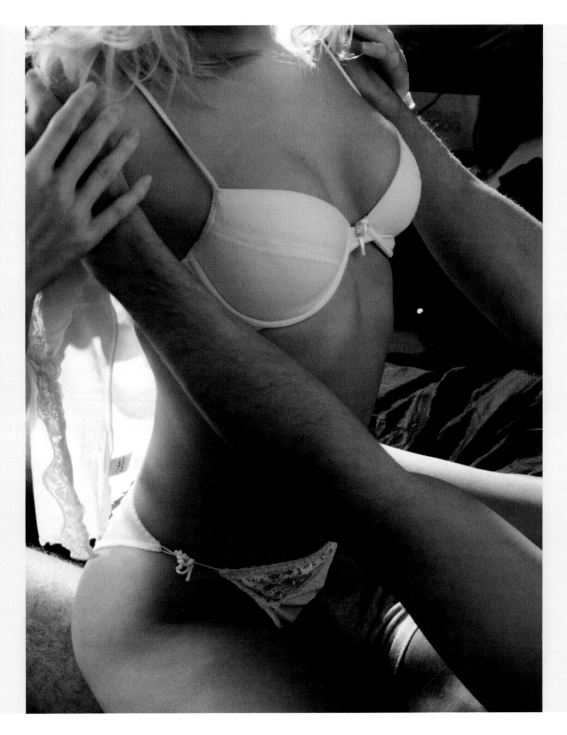

Wanting Less Sex Than Your Partner

The trouble with one partner not wanting as much sex as the other is that the other partner is constantly made to beg and plead. The supplicant begins to feel unloved, unattractive, angry and restless.

There's a variety of ways to work on this problem. If the less sexually active partner is willing, he or she might start using testosterone gel, rubbing it in to the skin on a regular basis on the grounds that this stimulates sex drive, arousal and sensitivity.

If the problem has arisen because the withholding partner is feeling steamrollered by his or her partner's needs, then a sex contract is useful. In this, you might mutually agree to you choosing for three nights of the week, your partner choosing for three nights of the week, and the seventh night can be up for grabs.

If the unwilling partner is bored, either by the sex or by the relationship, time needs to be spent talking. Can you make interesting enough conversation to rejuvenate sexual interest? Or can you decide to part on the grounds that you are unable to sustain a life with little or no sex?

MY MEME SUGGESTION

Be aware that marriages can survive without sex. It is your choice how you continue to be sexual. Other options include self-stimulation, another relationship or substitute hugs and cuddles.

Other ways you could think about it could include masturbating, enjoying sexual relationships outside your committed relationship, or simply getting so much hugging and cuddling from your committed partner that it largely makes up for the lessened penis/vagina contact. In case you doubt the possibility of surviving a marriage where sex is almost or completely gone, remind yourself that your doubts are based on a meme – the one that says you can't have marriage without sex. You can – and thousands do. Thousands of couples continue to love each other dearly enough to be able to give each other the freedom to be sexual in other ways.

Not Wanting Sex At All

This is an extended version of the previous problem.

If you both regret the loss of your love life, a medical examination might be in order. In the case of a male, Viagra, vacuum methods of sustaining an erection, or cutting down on the booze (alcohol creates impotence) might be solutions. If you are a female, take a look at what is happening to your hormones. Hormone supplementation might be a help.

If neither of you cares much about the continuity of sex, don't give it another thought. If you can manage to be happy without sex, good luck to you. You don't have a problem. But if one of you resents the situation, and the other doesn't, take a look at the answer to the previous question, including my meme suggestion.

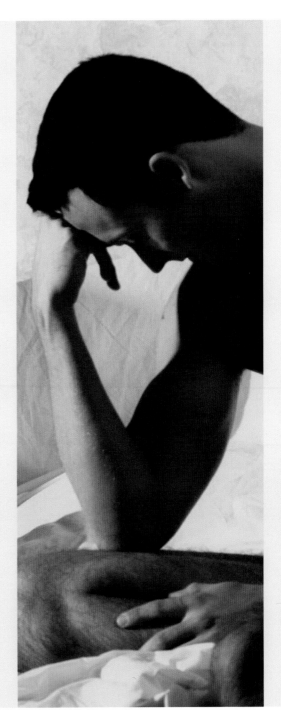

Getting Inhibited Because You Think You Ought to be Doing Sex Better

A typical example of this is a woman who believes she is spoiling her husband's enjoyment of sex because she isn't having orgasms. The more she will try to have orgasms under these conditions, the less likely it is that she will experience them. The more she attempts to loosen up her behaviour, the more threatening this will feel and the more inhibited she will become.

There are two areas to look at here. The easiest is to overcome the inhibition. If the couple works on giving each other sensual massage with intercourse forbidden, they can learn to progress to highly erotic massage in unpressurized circumstances. By doing this they may be able to educate themselves more accurately than they have previously managed about what it takes to get the woman through to orgasm. By combining the stimulus of erotic books or erotic films with self-massage, they may be able to successfully heighten the erotic atmosphere.

MY MEME SUGGESTION

Tell yourself that each one of us is responsible for our own orgasm. This means that if one person wants something improved it is up to that individual to improve it – not the partner.

Alternatively, this may be something the woman wants to do on her own in a programme of self-stimulation and self-exploration. (See the appendix for suitable training books.) The second area is the reason that the woman is feeling such anxiety in the first place. If her anxieties are based on the complaints of her partner, the problem may not be hers at all. Some men feel inadequate sexually and displace their feelings on to their wives. This may take professional counselling to improve.

On a purely practical level, this means that the dissatisfied partner needs to take a look at his own frustration. He is after all, managing to experience an orgasm. So what is it that doesn't work for him? If he is anxious about his skills as a lover, perhaps that ought to be the focus of marital counselling. If he has deep-seated anxieties about his effectiveness in the world, he needs to take a look at them. What he needs to be stopped from doing is dumping his anxieties on his partner. They do not belong to her.

CASE HISTORY

Anthony complained to me about his wife's lack of orgasm, describing her as frigid. Julia subsequently worked with me on learning to give herself an orgasm and managed it, without too much difficulty. It then became obvious that Anthony was a very poor lover who had never taken the trouble to stimulate his wife at all. When Julia went back into the relationship saying, 'Look, isn't it marvellous, I can climax. Let's do it together.' Anthony became impotent. He had felt powerful thanks to his assumed superiority. When he felt that superiority was taken away from him, he also felt threatened.

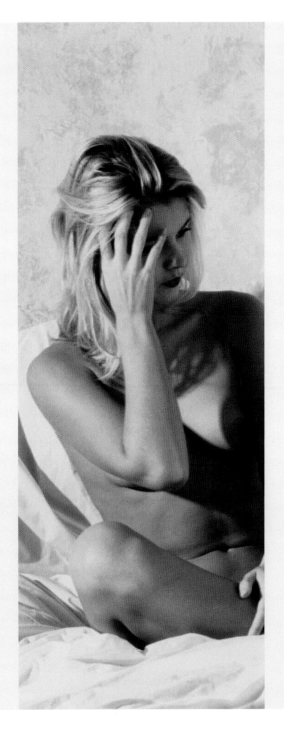

Finding it Hard to Start a Sexual Relationship

If you feel another person is expecting great things of you, and you know that you take your time in coming to the boil, this is an anxiety based on a belief about yourself. This belief says you have to be a perfect lover who makes no mistakes, and that if you cannot live up to this, then you are a failure as a person. You will be unable to hold on to a partner because you won't be attractive enough to retain his/her interest. And since you know you take time in which to get to trust someone and therefore to really let go sexually in his or her presence, you despair in advance.

Some of the messages of Assertion Training come in useful here. One of them is "It is OK to make mistakes but it's a good idea if you can learn from them". The whole point about mistakes is that they are half of a learning process. The other half is what you do with them. So, next time you meet a potential lover, explain at some appropriate stage that you need to take things slowly. Reveal that you get nervous because you fear too much will be expected of you too soon. If you feel that things are going too fast, don't hesitate to pull away. If your new partner moves too rapidly toward intercourse, pull back. Say, 'I really want to do this but I don't feel right about it yet.' Forty years of having a sex life have taught me that if your new partner is the 'right' one, he or she will understand and cope well, things will improve, and you won't compromise or freeze in fear. If your new partner is the wrong one, he or she won't have the patience to deal with your hesitations and you will have learned something valuable about him or her. If your partner can't be patient right at the start, he or she will be even less likely to be patient at any later stage.

MY MEME SUGGESTION

Recognize that the reason we persist with new partners who we fear may not be quite right, is because we fear we will never find one who is.

Learn to recognize and trust your instincts. Don't ditch people before you have given them a chance to unwind; after all, they may have the same difficulty as you. Give them time, and learn to feel good about yourself and your ability to survive without a partner if needs be. It is usually only when we have gained this kind of strength and independence that we become truly attractive. A common meme is that we cannot live without someone to love us. While it is certainly true that it much more pleasurable to love and be loved, you also can live perfectly happily without this. So reassemble your thoughts with regards your own inner strengths.

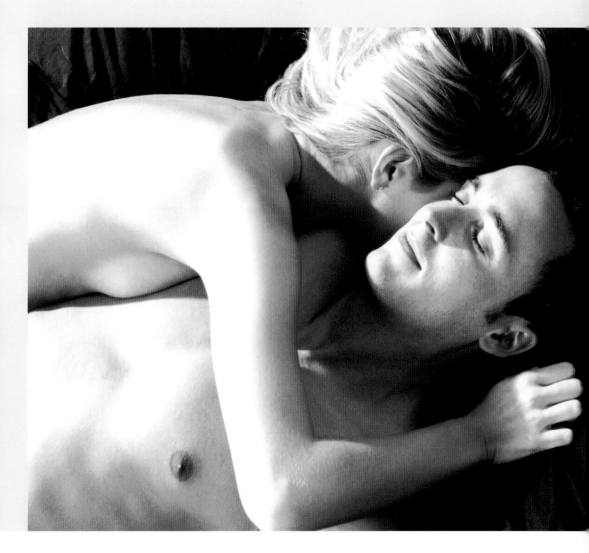

Feeling Inferior Because of Your Unconventional Sexual Ideas

If your idea of sex isn't doing it on a Saturday night in the marital bed in the missionary position, you are probably one of those lucky people with an effortless sexuality. It takes very little to make you come to orgasm, which means that you really adore going to that occasional 'special' party. You actually have experimented with threesomes and swinging – and lived to enjoy the experiences. But – and it's a big but – you are forced to keep completely quiet about your sexuality. You are quite sure that if you let on in any way about your sexual adventures, you will end up an outcast on the edge of society. And this has repercussions for married life.

It is almost impossible to settle down to the cosy routine of sex on a Saturday night because you just go mad with boredom and frustration. But you are a human being and you do want to settle down. So you feel very unhappy with yourself. You believe there is something intrinsically dirty about you and that you will never be good enough to deserve a regular marriage.

MY MEME SUGGESTION

Take a look at the prejudiced attitudes that say sex variations are wrong. See them for what they are – the mark of ignorance and fear.

This a heavy load to carry. You are presumably one of those people who is bold in bed but shy about expressing your independence of thought to a partner. Your instinct in not doing so may be entirely appropriate. But if a major force in your life has to be permanently hidden, it is indeed going to be difficult to find the right person to attach yourself to.

First of all, you must stop feeling inferior. You are as good and as valuable as anyone else. In some ways, you are blessed. There are great advantages to possessing an 'effortless sexuality'. You can be completely confident about this core part of your being, something that many others are not. Your sexuality is part of the normal range of human sexual response, and there is nothing wrong or 'dirty' about it or you. Your real problem is other people's judgmental ideas about your sexual behaviour. You don't want to be an outcast so just how do you proceed.

The answer would be to build on that 'easy sexuality' rather than shovel it under the carpet. The partner most likely to accept and appreciate you would be someone with a similar approach to life. Make relationships with people you meet at sex parties and give them the chance to continue outside the party. Start looking for emotional depths as well as sexual ones. Once you meet someone who can accept you, sexuality and all, you will start feeling much better about yourself.

When someone attacks sexual variety it is because he or she feels seriously threatened. There's no point in going around threatening people. Instead pay them the compliment of letting them keep their ideas but learn to be strong about your own. Yours are based on the knowledge that you are a perfectly decent human being. So, every time you get that inferior feeling back, tell yourself that it is someone else's fear that is trying to control you.

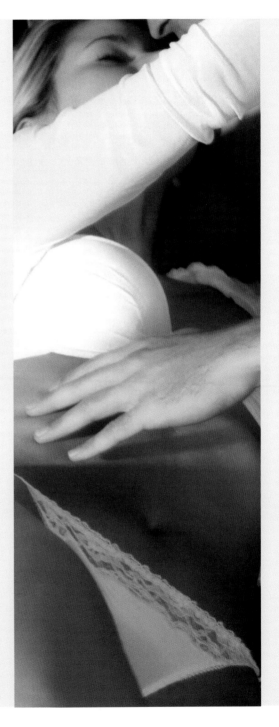

Feeling Inferior Because of Your Conventional Sexual Ideas

Every magazine you pick up has an article on how to do sex in 69 different positions. And you really don't like this. It's not that you begrudge other people hanging from a chandelier; it's just that you are getting to feel really inadequate because you never want to swing yourself. You enjoy sex all right but in its proper place. So how do you prevent yourself from feeling like 'Miss Conventionality'?

Derive comfort from the fact that although a lot is written about the newer raunchier sex lives of men and women, there's a big reality gap between the articles and real life. People like you are in the majority, so forget the publicity and look forward to Saturday night! If you want to make it special, give your partner a massage as a little extra. This is the friendliest, most sensual gift you can offer anyone. But, if you really don't want to do that, don't. You are entitled to your preferences.

MY MEME SUGGESTION

Next time a tinge of anxiety crosses your mind, remind yourself that most possible partners are likely to be highly relieved to know that you will settle for something regular but good.

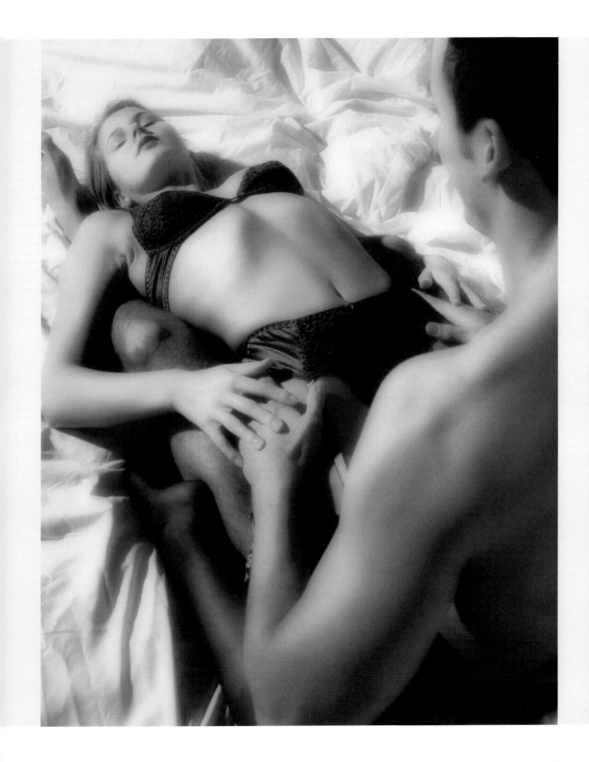

You Would Like to Experience Orgasm Every Time You Make Love

This doesn't always happen. Does this mean that something is wrong?

Not at all; desire is as variable as is the quality of orgasm. There are times when we make love only because our partner wants it. Even though we don't particularly feel like it, we go ahead because we love him or her. Sometimes there are other things on our mind that rob us of the ability to fully let go.

But what is important when this happens, is to explain why this has happened in such a way that your lover does not feel rejected. If, however, your lack of orgasm is happening more and more, then you need to take a look at yourself and how you are feeling about the relationship. What is happening to you or between you that seems to be putting orgasm out of the question?

MY MEME SUGGESTION

Understand that orgasm is variable, no female experiences it every time.

There is no 'correct' way in which to have sex. Of course, it is pleasant to experience orgasm but only if you really desire it. Desire is the crux – not orgasm. Nor is desire the only criterion. Just because you don't desperately desire someone sexually does not mean to say you don't love him or her. But it might mean that your relationship is changing in some way that needs to be acknowledged, if only by you.

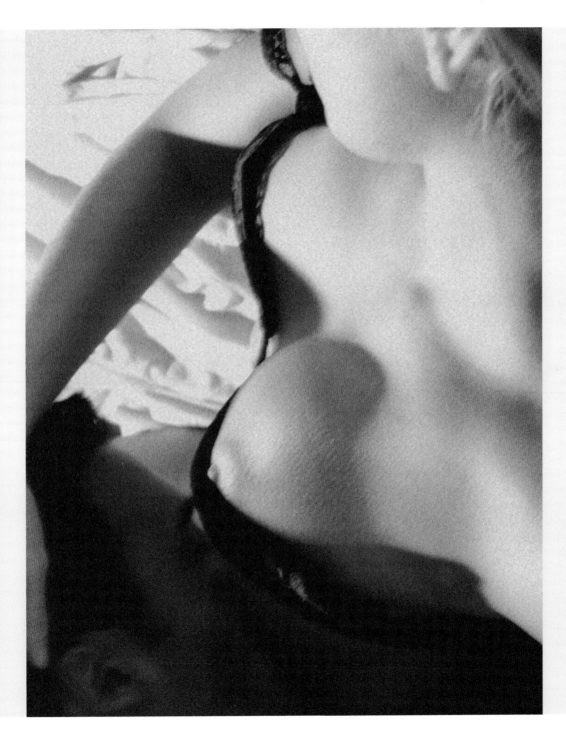

Feeling Unsatisfied by Your Orgasms

You are glad to have one at all but it seems short and slight. Why can't it be earth-shattering like in the romantic novels?

Orgasm is immensely variable. Not only does it vary from person to person but it also differs on nearly every occasion. If you haven't experienced an orgasm for a long time, it may be pent-up, explosive, strong, urgent and full of sharp sensation when it arrives. But if this is your fifth orgasm of the day, it may be difficult to attain, short, slight and with little or muted sensation.

Orgasm can go on for hours or it can last for a couple of seconds. Some people do not feel the sensation of their orgasm at all and only know it is happening because they feel the movement or watch the movement in a mirror – a kind of anaesthetized orgasm. Verbal descriptions of orgasm vary from

'It's like the gentle rippling of waves.'

to:

'It's a piercing sensation that spreads deeper and deeper until my whole body is sharp with amazing feeling.'

So why don't you experience something deeper? Here's a list of reasons.

MY MEME SUGGESTION

A glass half-empty is also a glass half-full. If none of my suggestions succeed, work on appreciating what you have got instead of lamenting what you don't have.

- You are not getting long enough erotic build up in advance. You need tons more foreplay that is delayed and delayed and delayed.
- If you are female, perhaps your partner is stopping stimulating you the minute your orgasm begins. Women differ slightly from men in that if the sensation is to continue for as long as possible, the clitoral sensation must continue too. Once it stops, so does the climax.
- You are so busy trying to control the orgasm that you and your body don't let go enough for the climax to feel really wild. You could try working on letting go. Try beating cushions, screaming, crying or shouting, especially when you feel yourself nearing climax.
- You've been having too much sex and each subsequent climax is harder to achieve and lessened in sensation. Lay off for a while and see what happens.
- If you are female, perhaps your hormone system is naturally a little short of free-ranging testosterone – the hormone that influences libido, desire and sensation. Try to find a specialist in sexual medicine who will assess your testosterone levels and, if appropriate, prescribe testosterone gel for you.
- If you are male, and if little or no sensation has always been the case, you may be suffering from insufficient testosterone or you may have some hang-ups that are affecting your mind control. The best way to sort this out is to get the various tests that tell you exactly where your hormone levels stand.
- Unless your orgasm is so slight as to be hardly felt, I would suggest you examine the relationship within which you are experiencing this difficulty. If the difficulty is with yourself, then you may need some medical assistance, but if it is only within the relationship that orgasm feels so unsatisfactory and if orgasm works fine during masturbation, then take a look at your feelings about exposing yourself sexually to this particular partner. Is it him or her particularly? Or is with every partner that this happens? It could be that you are suffering from one of the inhibition problems I mentioned earlier. You could work on these inhibitions with a therapist, which could help you to change some of the fixed ideas that are holding you back. If this doesn't work, you could try specific medication.

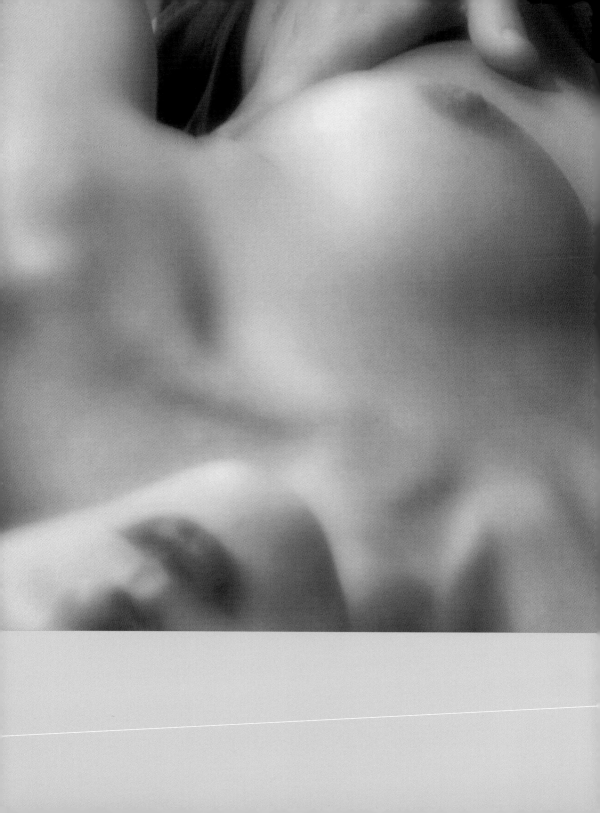

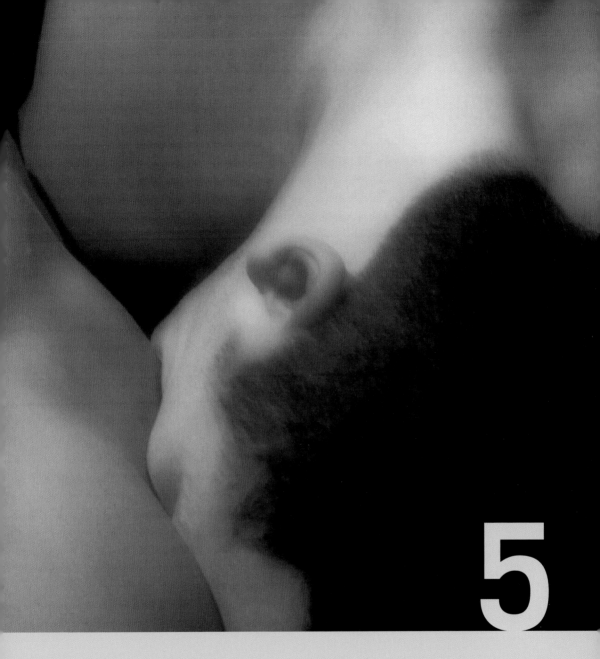

5

Sex Ideas Through Time

The Evolution Of Sex

The way in which we experience sex appears to change every couple of generations. There may not be a change in what actually happens (i.e. penis still goes into vagina), but there is a difference in how sex is seen and valued as an intrinsic part of life. Through thinking differently, the experience imperceptibly shifts. The computer generation, for example, used to taking on board short but sharp bursts of information, may need to experience sex much more hurriedly than former generations. We know this is already happening where reading is concerned. Concentration spans seem to be shortening but they are also becoming more intense.

In this section, we take a look at who we are sexually, bearing in mind that who we are depends on when we are. Our 'when' survey is limited to a little over 100 years, because it is only in the late 19th century that written records of sexual activities began to be kept.

But the sexual attitudes of our grandparents and great-grandparents are what we want to know about because it is these which have provided the building blocks of our sexual attitudes.

On the foundations of our grandparent's beliefs we build, renovate and recreate. We inherit some of their ideas and ways of being. But ways of thinking and being also evolve during our own time, thanks to the horizontal transmission of memes, the situation where we get ideas from our peers (our own generation), rather than solely from our parents. It can be a fascinating exercise to look back over the past century and work out what we may have taken on from our near ancestors and what we bring from our present-day culture.

The Late 1800s and the Early 1900s – The Double Standards

Undoubtedly in the Victorian days there were many fortunate men and women who hit upon good sexual experience by happy accident, just as there are today. But the overriding belief of middle-class Victorian men and women was that sex was not something nice, respectable women enjoyed. This was the age of such sexual repression that even the legs of chairs were covered up. Middle-class women did not expect anything ambitious in the shape of sexual ecstasy, indeed probably feared sexual encounters at the start of marriage and may have lived stoically without ever experiencing sexual pleasure. Working-class women, if wed to a poor and alcoholic husband, were highly likely to be used and abused by their menfolk. Since contraception was virtually non-existent, women in particular would have been desperate not to have sex so often because having sex also meant having yet another agonizing childbirth experience, another mouth to feed, even more exhaustion and yet more pressure.

Set against this was the double standard of the time, whereby men were believed to have uncontrollable sexual appetites, which had to be slaked for reasons of health. If you were a member of the middle class this meant you looked for sex with someone other than your nicely brought-up wife. In late Victorian times there were hundreds of thousands of prostitutes, women, boys and children. There were brothels in all the major cities, patronized by men who thought it normal to enjoy this alternative secret life. Enjoyable sex became something to hide, to be swept under the carpet. For wives, sex was irrevocably associated with child-bearing since even though methods of birth control existed, few 'nice' women knew about them.

Masturbation was looked on as physically harmful, with every teaspoon of semen equalling the loss of a pint of blood. Appalling contraptions were invented to circumvent the frequent and inveterate masturbator.

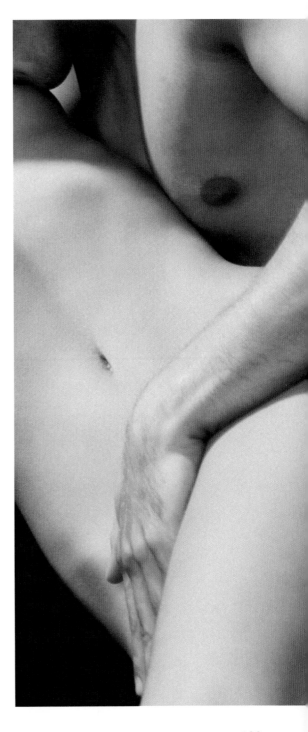

What might we have inherited from this?

The notions that sex:

- Should be hidden and never talked about;
- Can be responsible for poverty and starvation;
- In the shape of masturbation, is physically harmful and also that sex is dirty;
- Is only really enjoyable when done under 'forbidden' conditions;
- Is only really enjoyable when exploiting the vulnerable;
- Is a source of stress and conflict, misery and pain;
- Fine for men but out of the question for women.

The Other Victorian There was, however, one liberal feature of the late 1800s, and that was the work and translations by the great Victorian explorer Sir Richard Burton. Burton and his wife Isobel travelled extensively in Arabia and the Far East. Burton became fascinated by the ancient collections of erotic writing that he stumbled across. He commissioned English speakers amongst the native men to translate some of the books and published them by private subscription in England. He was so aware of the opprobrium he would generate by doing this that he chose to remain anonymous with the publication of the first book, the *Kama Sutra*. Word quickly got out, however, and he didn't bother to safeguard his anonymity with the publication of the next two, *The Perfumed Garden* and *The Ananga Ranga*. Although these were still most decidedly regarded as 'dirty books' there was nevertheless something exotic about them. They possessed a certain cachet, if only because Burton himself was a commanding figure and because eventually he did talk about them openly.

What we might have inherited from this?

The notions that sex might also

- Be exotic;
- Be a suitable interest for certain intellectuals and members of the upper classes, only provided that they were male, of course;
- Supply information about a variety of sex positions, and their particular strengths and weaknesses, or about matters of sexual etiquette and hygiene.

The 1920s and 1930s – Taking it to the Priest

Throughout the 19th and the early 20th century, there was a terrific rise in the power and role of the Church. Thousands of churches were built and attended, thanks to the prosperity of the time and social life that revolved around them. The priest was a pastor, the person to turn to in a time of trouble. Thanks to the devastation of the First World War (1914-1918), many social institutions and barriers broke down or dissolved and amongst these, to some degree, went the inhibition of talking about sex. It was during this period that the ideas of Freud, Jung and Adler reached a peak, and these and the combination of more conversation about sex (medical men thus setting an example), meant the breaking down of social taboos and that more and more men and women felt able to talk about their sexual problems. Though not, of course, with each other. This is where the priest came in. When men and women visited the priest for help, they didn't admit to having a sex problem. Their language was voiced in terms of faith. They presented their problems as spiritual ones.

It's important to make clear that up until now most nicely brought up women and many men simply knew nothing about sex. They didn't know how it worked, they knew nothing about female orgasm, they probably believed masturbation was harmful – there was an abyss of sexual ignorance. Growing out of the now greater discussion of sexuality came an awareness of the appalling living conditions of the working class as thanks to their enormous families. Marie Stopes and others began to set up the first birth control clinics to make contraception widely available and not just a luxury for those with money.

MARIE STOPES' POST BAG

Seeking spiritual help was particularly true of women. Marie Stopes, the British sexual and contraceptive reformer, received sackfuls of letters from distressed females after the publication of her highly controversial book *Married Love*. In these letters they regularly complained that they had consulted the priest about their pain or lack of enjoyment in the nuptial bed. By sorting out their spiritual life, it was explained, they would become easier and happier within themselves and their sexuality would be that much more likely to flow smoothly. In the sense that this is a forerunner of psychosexual counselling, there is truth in this. However practical help in the shape of physical work and medical intervention was a long way off still. Stopes' letters told of truly bleak marriages. In the US, Margaret Sanger did similar pioneering work on sexual reforms such as birth control.

What might we have inherited from this?

The notions that sex can be:

- Talked about;
- Controlled;
- Understood;
- Enjoyed by women provided they have the right education.

But also that teaching and education about sex was inherent to the Church and more directly the ministers.

The 1940s and 1950s – Sex Becomes Medicalized

Thanks to the growing availability of birth control for women, sex slowly began to become medicalized. During war time men had been able to talk to their medical officer about any sexual problems mainly as a precaution given to the forces with regards to controlling venereal disease. Once the Second World War was over, women began to talk to their doctors about birth control and gynaecological problems – not, however, about what actually happened between man and woman in bed. Since the help available was confined to health matters this meant that physical health improved, but the actual nitty gritty of what went on between the sheets did not. Nice men and women still did not talk openly about sex, thanks to their Victorian inheritance. The result of this is that there were still a lot of misconceptions. Women were generally believed to have no equivalent sexual response to that of men because they were not capable of ejaculation. Many doctors believed (and continued to do so until the 1980s) that, because of this, women did not climax or at least experienced only an incomplete and inferior orgasm. This meant that men could feel supremely confident about their own sexual performance but often, unfortunately, at the expense of their partner.

What might we have inherited from this?

The notion that:

- Sex is a medical issue but still not to be talked about outside the marriage bed;
- Women are sexually inferior to men and unlikely to have any kind of equivalent response;
- Men must be responsible for women's lesser sexuality;
- Women must be shown what to do.

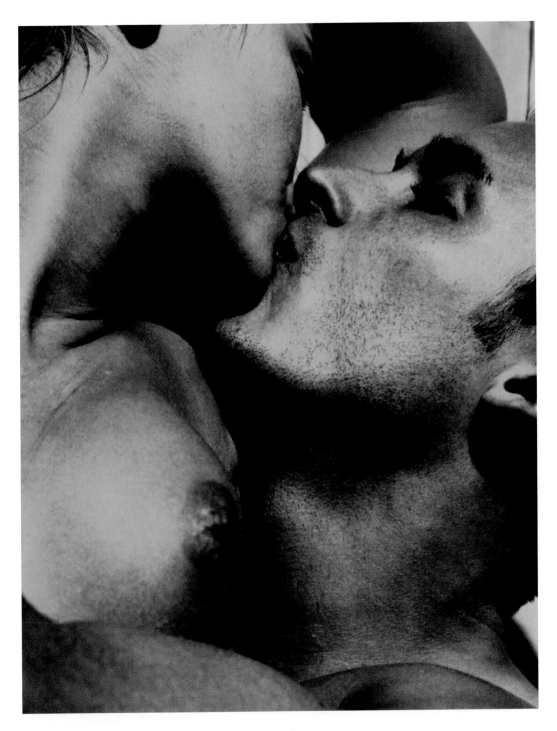

The 1960s to the 1980s – Taking it to the Relationship Counsellor

This was an era of flowering sexual research. Thanks to the pioneering work done by Alfred Kinsey and Masters and Johnson in the 1940s and 1950s, the new information filtered through to the general public slowly but surely during the 1960s and 1970s. Men and women learned that they might expect major changes in their most intimate life.

Men learned that they might to some extent control certain sex problems instead of feeling helpless about them. Women learned that not only were they not sexually inferior but that thanks to multiple orgasm they might be superior. Suddenly, orgasm became a possibility for everyone. There was the bonus that everyone talked about it. But now different pressures settled on male and female shoulders. Men complained that women were too demanding. Thanks to the growth of feminism and the relative safety of the contraceptive pill, women were suddenly unafraid to ask for more satisfactory sex and were no longer prepared to put up with poor-quality delivery. This put huge pressures on to men. The relationship between the sexes became over-sexualized. You were supposed to have sex often in the name of normality.

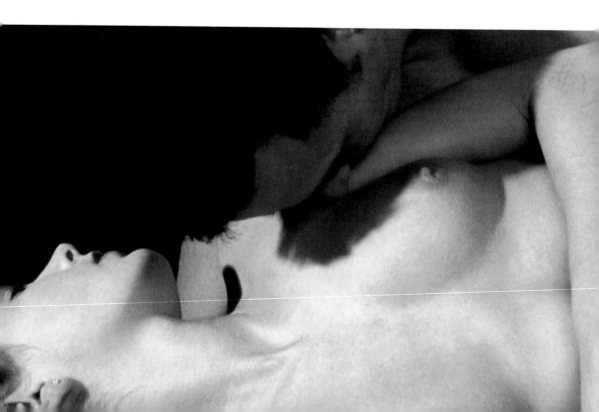

Since having sex all the time was easier said than done, people began to need a lot reassurance. The role of the relationship counsellor was invented, and instead of continuing to go to the priest with your spiritual dilemma, you visited the therapist with your sexual dilemma instead.

What might we have inherited from this?
We may believe that:

- A good sex life is everyone's right and that we can all expect to enjoy a lot of orgasms in our time;
- Women can be just as potentially dynamic in bed as men and that this is normal – it doesn't mean that they are somehow 'bad' people;
- Thanks to effective birth control, we no longer need to choose sexual relationships so carefully since we are unlikely to bear babies as a result. Recreational sex can be one of our pastimes.

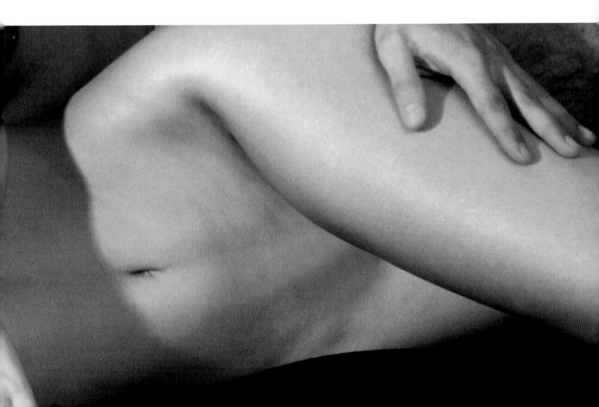

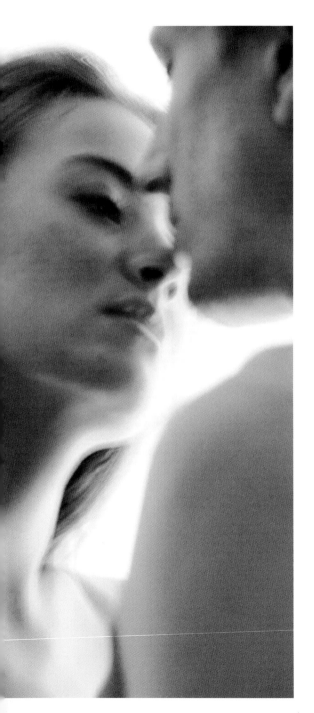

The 1990s – A Swing to the Pharmaceutical

By the end of the 1990s, a great deal of work had been carried out on the physiology of sex – how sex actually works. While during the 1970s, 90 per cent of sex problems were considered to be all in the mind, now the balance swung to the belief that at least 66 per cent of sex problems are caused by physical dilemmas. All that was needed was to pop a pill and hey presto – off you go again. Human beings learned to chemically modify their ability to function. And went to considerable expense in order to do so. But by now the hype about sex had become so extreme that another belief emerged – if you didn't enjoy sex, you didn't possess a personality. It thus became imperative that sex worked and was seen to work. This was in spite of pretty consistent surveys, which showed that up to half of men and women having regular sex considered that there to be something unsatisfactory about it, which probably indicates that it is normal for sex to vary enormously in quality.

What might we have inherited from this?

Many people now believe that:

- Sex works mechanically;
- You can have ultimate control over sex;
- You should be able to have sex with anyone and enjoy it;
- You can fix anything.

In The New Millennium

Drugs continue to be an overriding interest with longevity drugs keeping people younger and testosterone gel endowing men and women with a prolonged ability to feel and respond sexually. But the scientific emphasis is shifting gradually to understanding how the brain works. It is no accident that this book is written in terms of evolution, and in particular, of how our brains function and how we may or may not be able to programme our little grey cells. It is on the basis of a greater understanding of how the brain controls the body that we may get to consciously think differently (or alternatively) about sex. One observation about the role of testosterone in sexual function has been to make a connection between increased sexuality and enhanced imagination. It would be interesting if, on this basis, creativity turned out to be irrevocably linked to sexual dynamism. In the next section I talk about possible connections between the two and how we may bring creativity into day-to-day sexual fun.

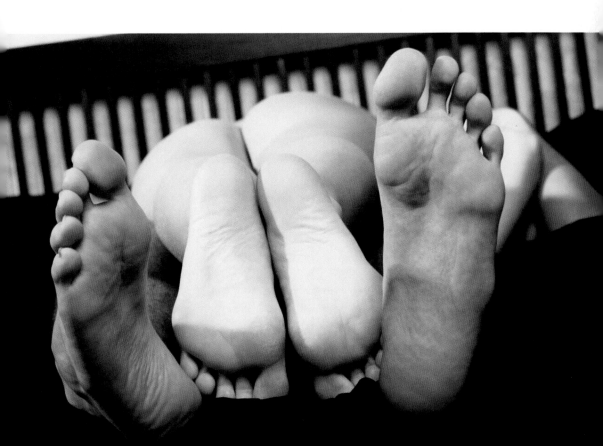

Looking Back

After re-reading this section you may perceive that many of the beliefs we have inherited from our forebears are in conflict with each other. Most of us believe the old ideas and the new ones. We can probably see, with all our considerable acuity, that one custom makes a great deal of sense and yet, for some intangible reason, we cannot subscribe to it. What holds us back? Almost certainly it is great-grandmother, lodged defiantly inside our 21st century brain. Take just one contemporary belief – that we ought to be able to let go and enjoy sexually with any halfway suitable partner. Our great-grandmother will tell us that we are immoral creatures for wanting to do this, that we somehow defile ourselves, and even though we now think this to be rubbish, the idea is there, inside, directing the traffic of our thoughts. It also gets clearer as we look back that many of the beliefs were erroneous in the first place. This means it is perfectly possible that we, in the here-and-now, are still functioning on misbelief. It's another reason why we need to look deeper into our murky sexual psyches.

How Can You Identify the Sexual Beliefs of Your Own Family?

It helps to have living elderly relatives whom you could talk to. Contrary to what you might expect, many of these elders are interested in looking back and identifying the origins of how they themselves lived their own long lives.

Without being overly prurient, you can garner a surprising amount of information (see questions, opposite), which gives a good idea of how your near ancestors lived their sexual lives. Look out for dramatic incidents such as unwed parenthood, rejection by parents, a secret abortion, a jilted or jilting lover, an alcoholic partner who sexually terrorized, war time disability that affected a sex life, the list is endless. These are all events, which will in some tiny way impact on your own life today. Now make a list of your own sexual beliefs (see Chapter 4) and see if you can link these to the events you have just researched

QUESTIONS FOR ELDERLY RELATIVES

- What was the relationship like between their parents?
- What religious beliefs might have directed them?
- What social background did they emerge from and how might have this impacted on their beliefs?
- What were the circumstances of their early lives? Did they grow up in times of peace or of war?
- Were they rich or poor?
- Did their parents seem loving towards each other?
- How many children did they have?
- Did they themselves ever suffer from and repressive social attitudes about sex?
- Did they have an enjoyable physical relationship with their own partner or were there difficulties?

The Family Constellation

Another exercise, borrowed from Adlerian psychology, is to picture your family as a constellation of stars. See yourself as the sun, which, of course, is the biggest brightest star, and place each member of your family either close or far, depending on what you feel is his or her influence on you. When you have drawn up your constellation, take a look at the characters who are closest and think about the sexual example that they may have provided. What might you have unconsciously learned from these emotionally close relatives about sensuality?

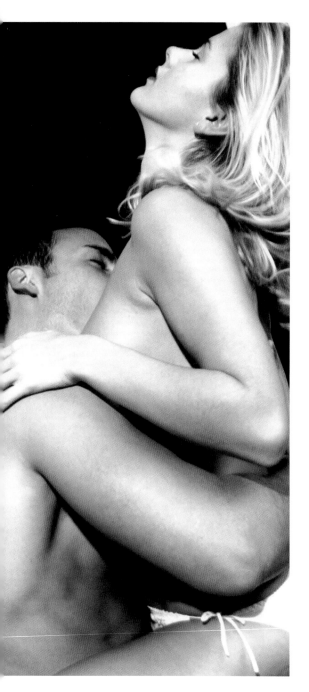

Identify the Snapshot

How might you identify the way in which you yourself are likely to approach sexuality and in particular, sexual problems? Think back to your earliest childhood. Remember the earliest incident regarding sexuality that comes to mind. Now picture this incident as a scene in a film. Next, freeze the frame of the film so that you are just looking at a static picture. What title would you give the picture? And what feelings does this special scene evoke? See the example, opposite.

If underlying feelings about sex are unconscious you might ask: why bother to find out what they are? The reason for doing so is that by becoming aware of unconscious motivation, it brings your actions and behaviour into the conscious. You can then consciously choose to alter your sexual behaviour if that is what you prefer. Or you can continue to sin with impunity!

The methods just described work even more effectively when both members of a couple identify their unconscious feelings about sex and then compare notes. Anna found that her partner's feelings led him to be assertive about the way in which he carried out his sex life. She loved this because his ready expectation that any sex was good sex overcame her feelings of guilt. It also suited the defiant aspect of her character in that it allowed her to be more sexual than her inner grandmother would have liked.

Anna's Story

Film scene.

'One of my earliest memories is of playing sex games with another little girl at about the age of eight. The door to my room opens and in comes my grandmother who is not pleased to find out what we are doing. In future, the little girl and I are not allowed to play with each other any more and although I didn't feel at the time as if I was doing anything wrong, now I feel guilty. Somehow, unknowingly, I was bad.'

Snapshot.

'I am halted mid-game, with my grandmother's face peering around the door.'

Title of snapshot.

Bad Girls

Feelings.

'I've disgraced myself but I don't know why.'

Possible impact on future.

It may be hard for Anna to trust either her own feelings or those of a new partner since there now exists this awful underlying feeling that she might be disgracing herself all over again. Alternatively, she might be so angry about feeling guilty that she becomes defiant. Her reaction, therefore, might be to become blatantly and defiantly sexual. This is not to say that any of these feelings work on a conscious level. But they may underpin everything about her sex life at an unconscious level.

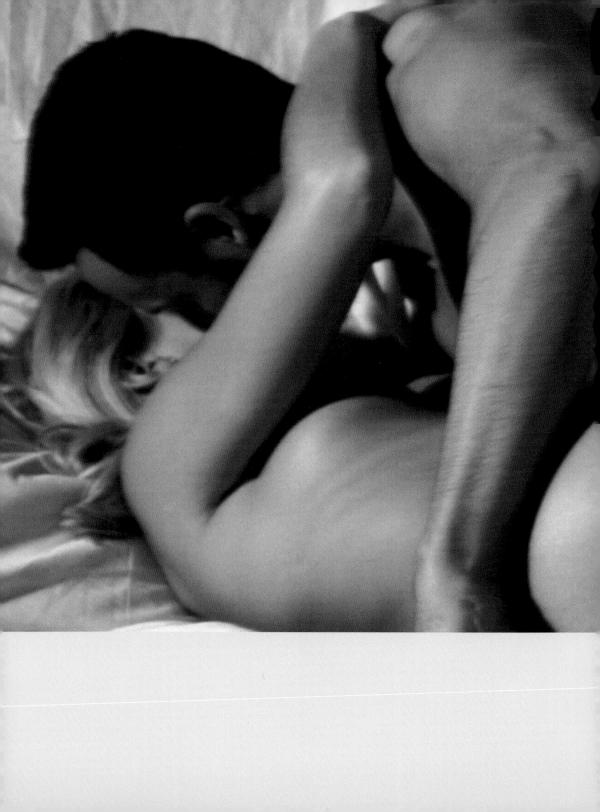

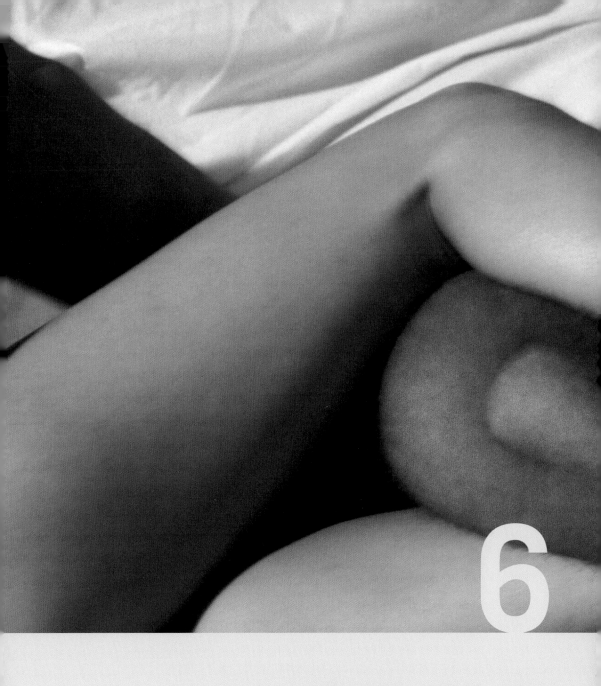

6

Sex as Creativity

The Energetic Nature of Sex

The link between sex and creativity is energy. One of the early explanations of the creation of the world believed that the world was the result of a cataclysmic orgasm of the gods – a fusion of sex and energy. Yet in all the subjective descriptions of sexuality we are currently presented with, little attention has been paid to the fact that, not counting conception, the sex act is an intensely creative event. It is perhaps one of the most creative actions that human beings ever perform.

When we begin having sex, we don't actually know how to do it. We understand the functions but we don't know how to do the feelings, the approaches, when and where to lay our hands. We do not usually have other people set an example or teach us. We are forced to come up with a way of doing sex all by ourselves that is uniquely and creatively our own. It is particularly creative because it is an invention of not one but two people and as such the permutations are multiplied – there may be many wonderful variations of such an invention. And, for ever afterwards it remains creative because every experience of sex is a new experience. Each time we do sex, we are a day older, we think differently, we move differently, we bring a different mood to our coupling.

Freud's Legacy

Sex has been linked to many sorts of creativity other than the sex act – albeit often in a negative way. One of Freud's legacies has been to see sex as a cause of envy, a reason for sublimation, a target for repression, although not all of the blame should be laid at his door. Freud was probably only echoing the sexual sentiments of his time. As a result, writers, artists, philosophers and anyone making any kind of original movement in their life, were subsequently thought to be either:

- Compensating for some lack they felt (left over from childhood);
- Defending themselves from something bad, either real or imagined;
- Rewarding themselves in fantasy because real life is ultimately not rewarding;
- Sublimating infantile sexuality.

Possibly all of these suggestions regarding creativity are true. Yet these are only a part of the picture. It is like observing that the glass is half-empty. If you take the view that the glass is half-full, you get to see there are many highly positive links between creativity and sex as well.

When Sex Involves Play

Sexual creativity comes in many forms. One form is play. People play. They play at all stages of their life and they particularly play in bed. Yet there have been difficulties in understanding what evolutionary survival value play possesses. One argument has it that play allows you to rehearse situations. Yet other thinkers have pointed out that it is not necessary to play in order to rehearse. Another argument has it that play is a simple physical release of energy. Yet there are many ways in which to release energy without involving the fun aspect.

Watching animals at play you can see the difference between play behaviour and serious behaviour. According to psychiatrist Anthony Storr, play behaviour is exaggerated and uneconomical. The motor patterns used in play are those which the animals might use in serious situations but they are used in the wrong order, or done incompletely or repeated over and over again, or exaggerated so that they are inefficient. And it's the same with humans. What's more, higher animals such as the primates, most especially the chimpanzee, can extend play to such skills as painting pictures with oil paints. According to zoologist Desmond Morris, chimpanzees become so absorbed in painting that they sometimes have tantrums when they are stopped. They may prefer painting to feeding, and as a result get caught up in what Desmond

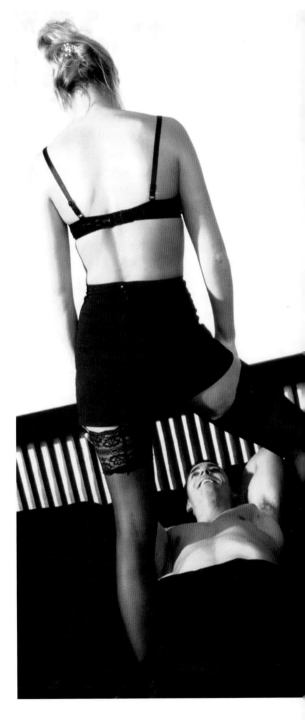

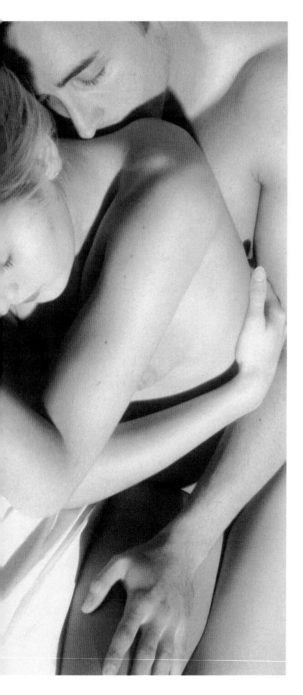

calls 'self-rewarding activities'. Most aspects of sex are also self-rewarding – I doubt if there are many individuals who only do sex for the sake of others. And, of course, we play during sex. We endlessly create and recreate our expressions of love and sensuality. We reward our partners by doing so. We reward ourselves. Just as writing a book is tangible evidence of creative 'play', the sense of connection between lovers is intangible evidence.

Sexual creativity and 'survival' Desmond Morris considers play to be an 'extra', something done for its own sake. Yet the human being who can play and be creative in entertaining a mate, may pull in a better mate than the human who is not. Play (and the arts linked with play) may well give us evolutionary survival advantages.

But what about survival in the here and now? The most obvious advantage to sexual play and to the creative arts is that both safeguard against boredom. If you think that boredom is irrelevant to survival please think again. Emotional survival in human beings is as almost as important as physical survival. If we have nothing left to live for we tend to die.

(Hu)Man requires constant stimulation Desmond Morris explains that there is a physical underpinning for such a notion. He says man and the higher primates belong to a category of animal that requires constant stimulation if the nervous system is to function at its most efficient. If there isn't any immediate stimulation from the surroundings, then the creature or human will seek out something or invent it. It sounds as if in order to continue 'being' we have to continue 'doing' or, at the very least, 'experiencing', even if it is at second-hand. To term experiences through art as 'second-hand' is a misnomer, however. We only ever experience life through the medium of our own brain. Any experience in the brain therefore is of direct value.

If we bring these ideas back to sex, and if we return to some of Freud's premises, it becomes apparent that sexual play is not just an infantile approach, or a rehearsal or a method of learning. Taken to its heights, sex can be viewed as the ultimate projection of pure self – a true sexual creation. And people adore the experience of sexual creation because that pure self feels so good. The pleasure and joy of good sex between two loving people feels as though something tangible and ecstatic is created. In the physicality of sex, brilliant, scintillating emanations charge the air with positive energy.

When the cup is half-full

So we might also be able to view sexual creativity as:

- Enlarging on and remembering valuable experience;
- Opening up to good experiences, either real or imagined;
- Sharing with the community the artist's (or lover's) own valid life experience;
- Celebrating life in the shape of sexuality.

One of the reasons why Freud may have worked out only half the picture is because he left an important ingredient out of his version of psychology, which his rival and contemporary Alfred Adler thought to include. This ingredient is the need to feel connected to others, something that Adler called *gemeinshaftsgefuhl* or translated, 'human interest'. It is that sense of connectedness that enables us to revel in wonderful sex, to long to share good feelings with others, and to use the media of writing, painting and music to do precisely that.

How Sexual Dilemmas Can Be Seen Positively

That's all very well you may say, but right now my sexual experiences are negative. How do I turn my sexuality around so that I read it as though the cup is half-full?

One approach is to look for important messages that your behaviour or lack of behaviour is offering. If you work from the premise that all behaviour has meaning, even behaviour that is termed 'bad', this makes the way that you live your sex life fascinating. If you can identify what your behaviour (or the behaviour of a partner) is telling you, you enrich your being. If all behaviour has meaning this means that there is no negative behaviour, just meaningful behaviour. By seeing your sex life as a form of creativity you gain a new perspective on it – however 'good' or' bad' you consider it to be.

To give you an idea of how to do this, I am going to turn the tables on three sexual situations that are commonly defined as types of moral dilemma. I will attempt to interpret these dilemmas creatively.

1. When you have sex with someone you hardly know.

The negative interpretation is that sex with strangers is immoral and that no 'nice' person would have sex with someone they've only just met. Such an action tends to be viewed as the behaviour of someone desperate, over-needy, exploitative, reckless or feckless. All of which may be true. But it leaves out a lot of other explanations, all of which are equally valuable.

A method of 'getting-to-know-you'

The positive interpretation says that even if you are having sex with someone you hardly know, sex can be the start of a process of showing this new person a special, inner you. And this can be true, regardless of who the partner is, be he or she prostitute, swinger or simply new friend.

A method of 'getting-to-know-yourself'

What's more, sex is also a process of showing you the inner you. How else can you know what you are like in differing sexual circumstances except to experience them? The difference between you and others (who do not act similarly) is that you have the courage to experiment where they do not.

A childhood method of emotional survival

How you first get to know someone sexually may be due to the kind of emotional survival beliefs you developed while you were growing up. If you were starved of love and affection in formative years you may not only be needy for these in adulthood, you may be greedy, too. Your unconscious may have figured out that if you don't grab it as soon as it's available, you may not get the chance again. 'Go for it and don't waste time on the preliminaries,' is what your inner child is telling you. Your internal logic is trying to protect you against isolation and desolation. And sex is commonly misunderstood by many of us to be love and affection.

Your unconscious here is working on the survival patterns that it learned in infancy. But when we work things out for ourselves as little children we sometimes get things wrong. Or even if we didn't get it wrong at the age of four, it may not actually be relevant 20 years later. So although sex with complete strangers may feel instinctively comforting at one level, such a direct approach may bring as many problems as solutions.

Accepting your direct approach

Fortunately, gaining such an insight can be used in many ways. You may decide that you are happy with your direct approach to sex and that this is your own, very personal method of getting to know someone. The sex act can indeed act as a shortcut, assisting you to know someone on an inner level. You can learn things from sex. You can discover, from the way another expresses him- or herself, whether he or she is tender, abrupt, thoughtful, selfish. All of this information can be seen in body language, through verbal skills, as a result of eye movements. In the short space of a 15-minute encounter, you can understand if you really want to develop a relationship with this person or not.

As long as the other person can deal with this, such an approach can turn into a loving and enduring relationship. I know couples who met through going to swinging parties. Their first introduction was during sexual intercourse. By puritanical standards, they should have gone

LOOK FOR THE POSITIVE ASPECTS

We have consciously looked here at the positive side of the dilemma. Anyone can do the same. And there are good reasons for opening your mind to positive types of sexual approaches. If you tell people that something is wrong with them, this approach is supremely unhelpful. Not only is any advice rejected out of hand, but enough additional anger may be engendered to compound the behaviour. On the other hand, looking for and finding out what is relevant works. Men and women listen, they feel good, they feel relaxed enough to take in any constructive approaches subsequently put forward. When they can feel that a sexual choice is their own and not something foisted upon them, they then reach a position where they can take the responsible option that properly suits them, rather than what suits the person who is advising.

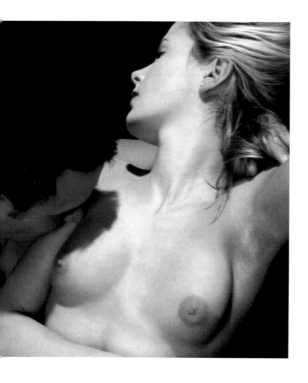

straight to hell, not passed God and definitely not have been able to score a bull's-eye with a new relationship. Yet they liked each other so much that they started dating. They carried out courtship backwards and ended up moving in together. If you can manage to lose the judgemental attitudes that you were almost certainly brought up with, you begin to see that there are many distinct possibilities for life that cannot be taken on board by a rigid and inflexible mind.

Moderating your direct approach

On the other hand, you may feel that your instant tendency to jump into bed is beginning to harm you. You may prefer to slow your sex life down a bit but find it difficult to do because all your instincts goad you to do otherwise. Trying not to have sex can surprisingly feel risky – as though you will be rejected, as though nobody will like you, even as if you may never find a partner. This is a tough set of feelings to overcome. But... it can be done! There are several methods of moderating the anxiety you feel when you draw back from instant sex.

Next time you find yourself about to bundle into bed, stop for a minute, remove yourself to the bathroom and look at your face in the bathroom mirror. Now repeat the mantra 'I AM OK WITHOUT SEX' several times.

If you still find yourself zipping off to the nearest king-size, look at the fingers on your right hand and wiggle them one by one as you repeat the mantra.

Next, tell your partner that you think he or she is gorgeous but you do not yet feel comfortable with them. Suggest instead that you meet for a further date because 'you would really like to get to know them better'. If the new friend is going to be halfway suitable they will play ball with this suggestion. If they don't, they are wrong for you – not you for them. And any time you feel a resurgence of that anxiety, wiggle the fingers of your right hand, and say 'I AM OK WITHOUT SEX'.

If the anxiety still persists, think of something you really like, such as a pair of favourite shoes and go straight to the wardrobe and put them on. By substituting a mantra, or your favourite shoes for your needy anxiety activity, you will start to feel better. Finger-wiggling sounds daft but it's a simple version of strategic therapy.

2. Sex with yourself.

How often have you heard the words 'Oh, he's a sad wanker'? Part of our Victorian inheritance is to believe that there is something weak, harmful or immature about masturbation. Anthony Storr, for example, in his book *The Dynamics of Creation*, states that self-stimulation acts as a short circuit because instead of relating to the real world, it throws the masturbator back on himself and effectively short circuits sex's connection with real life. His conclusion is that the masturbator is unlikely to produce any serious works of art because all his imagination will be channelled into his masturbation.

A logical approach

Let's take a closer look at this self-rewarding sexual activity. Storr might also add, if continuing to argue logically, that masturbation must also prevent the masturbator from making any serious relationship since his imagination would still be channelled elsewhere. But (unless someone is a complete obsessive), this is nonsense. You might just as well argue that someone with a full heterosexual love life couldn't be a great writer or composer either – sexual intercourse occupying the same creative space as masturbation. Yet we are certain that this is nonsense. Picasso is an obvious example of a great creator who thoroughly enjoyed sex. Mozart is another. Both intercourse and masturbation require energy and imagination and logically neither is a bar to creativity.

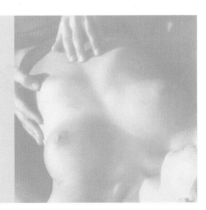

USE EMPATHY

In this dilemma, I have suggested putting yourself into the other person's shoes to get a true idea of his or her motivation. Learning to be empathic prevents us from becoming overly me-centred and lets us see all sides of a problem instead of only an entrenched or paranoid one.

The celebratory approach

I would see masturbation to be an extension of pure self – a method of expressing 'being', just as I would also see great art functioning in the same way. Far from any of these activities being sublimations, they can be wonderful methods of keeping in touch with your self-value, self-confidence and inner beauty. We all like to think we are OK individuals. Masturbation is a basic, primitive and pure method of so doing. Instead of turning us inwards, masturbation can equip us for handling the world with equanimity.

Masturbation develops the imagination

But masturbation is more than an expression of 'being'. It is a training-ground for the body, for getting to know your sexual response, for taking charge of your own sexuality. It offers information, which can be brought into a relationship with a lover so that you can both feel unpressurized. Masturbation is a method of developing the imagination. It is a rescuer. It rescues its happy practitioners from a lack of sensuality, from sexual frustration and from boredom. It is a healer; it comforts in times of sadness, and feels good at times of quiet.

When should you stop someone from masturbating?

A common sex problem focuses on the discovery by a loving wife that her husband is regularly masturbating. She reacts by feeling terribly hurt. She interprets his actions as meaning she is not enough for him. She may possibly be right. But she may also be completely wrong. If she interprets his actions from his point of view and not hers, she might find many perfectly innocent alternatives. For example, he may be masturbating from time to time purely because he likes it. And why shouldn't he? You don't usually prevent a partner from eating chocolates, do you? You understand his preference because you like chocolate too. In fact, you are probably glad he is having a great time feasting his taste buds.

It is possible to look on masturbation in the same non-judgemental way as chocolate-eating. One way of doing so is to keep an eye out for the positive aspects. What are those? The positive sides to masturbation are that the masturbator probably has:

- A high sex drive;
- A versatile sexual imagination which you, as his partner, are lucky enough to benefit from when the two of you do enjoy sexual intercourse.

We don't own our partners even though sometimes we would like to. They are separate people, who, if we are lucky, will enjoy journeying through life side by side with us. One of the hardest tasks in marriage is to tolerate each other's differences. Attitudes to masturbation may be one of these. His attitude may be quite different to yours. So the secret is to detach yourself from your territorial instincts, cut out any suspicion that your partner's masturbation may reflect on you, and look instead for his or her true inner motivation.

3. Sex is an ecstatic experience.
This is a moral dilemma in reverse. Although many people would like to believe such a premise, it is often seen as an empty one – the by-product of trashy romantic novels. Alternatively, certain religious movements teach that the only true ecstatic experience is that of oneness with God. So the concept of ecstatic sex is, for some people, a hot potato.

An orgasm is … just an orgasm.
And very nice, too! But very occasionally, by accident we get a glimpse of another reality. And one way of doing so is through sex. It's the white light, the blinding flash, the projection out into a cool bright space, where for seconds only, you experience pure ecstasy. And it does exist. It isn't just a figment of Barbara Cartland's imagination. But we have learned to distrust such an experience, to think of it as unreal, of no account, as some kind of fantasy put out into the ether by strange and ancient gurus.

Who's got time for spirituality?
We no longer associate ecstasy (of any sort) with our hurrying, scurrying 21st century lives. We

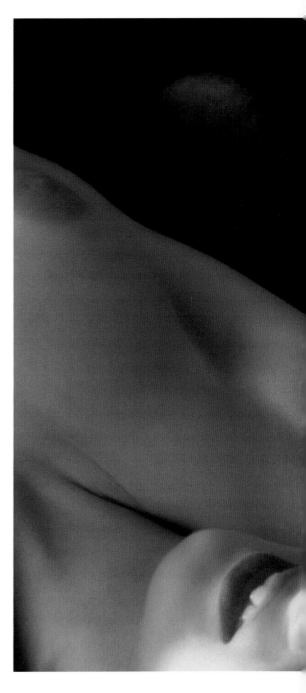

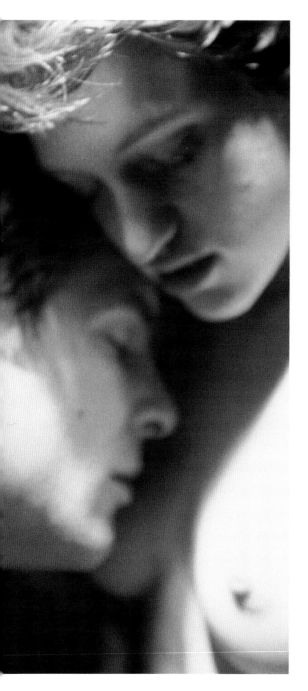

certainly don't want to credit sexual ecstasy as a serious possibility because if we do, we may have to acknowledge that there is something we haven't got, something missing. We are enormously grounded in today's reality, in the here-and-now. A spiritual life, of any sort, is considered something for earlier generations, but too fusty for most forward-thinking contemporaries. Apart from which, who's got the time?

And yet ... If we think like this we may be defending ourselves from disappointment but we will also be limiting our possibilities. The edge to the kind of excitement termed ecstasy is a sense of true connectedness; there's an impression that through the amazing well-being which flashes across the brain we can somehow share that well-being; that if one of us experiences it, so too, can anyone else. Even if this is an illusion, it is a particularly marvellous one. I have no doubt that the more of us who manage to suffer such an illusion, the better.

Have strength – think spiritual

So I would like to put in a plea for at least considering the possibility that sexual ecstasy exists. I don't believe it is something we can experience very often. But the occasional fleeting glimpse is wonderful. I'm not even sure that any of the disciplines designed to lead towards it will actually work. But if you analyse the ingredients of such disciplines, there's an emphasis on time, peace, unhurried sensuality, thinking and sharing. All of those are valuable.

You are right if you think there is nothing particularly new about sexual ecstasy. Ancient belief systems have taught it for thousands of years. It's what Tantric sex is all about. Yet my guess is that the notion of sexual ecstasy upsets certain moralists. If everyone were busy aiming at white lights and pure peace, wouldn't the world go mad? Wouldn't it spiral out of control, upsetting all the great institutions that have ruled for the last 2,000 years? So, in order to avoid such moral chaos, the idea of sexual ecstasy has been quietly relegated to a backwater. It takes faith to persevere with an idea that has been downgraded. Nevertheless a return to some of the old beliefs, bringing to them the benefits of new technical knowledge, often helps us make leaps of understanding.

Tangling with Tantra

Those who are keen to explore sex in the brain might consider buying copies of the *Kama Sutra* or invest in Tantric sex manuals. Alas, the observation of a certain ritual does not, unfortunately, ensure that you will reach heaven. And yet, who knows? Perhaps you might. Much of what the manuals teach makes sense. To repeat, the ingredients of Tantric sex are time, relaxation, the cultivation of extreme intimacy, the slow, gradual build-up of desire and tactile sensation. If you follow this advice, you achieve a type of timelessness. And when sexual excitement and orgasm become timeless that's when ecstasy sets in.

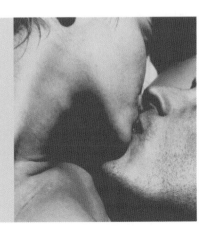

HAVE FAITH IN YOUR INSTINCTS

If you honestly believe that you have been lucky enough to clock out to a Karmic universe before arriving back on the bed in a tangle of sheets and duvets, don't be afraid. Explore this belief. It can't hurt anyone and it sure as hell, beats cocoa for a bedtime experience. It is by considering and measuring our gut emotions that we enable ourselves to grow emotionally strong.

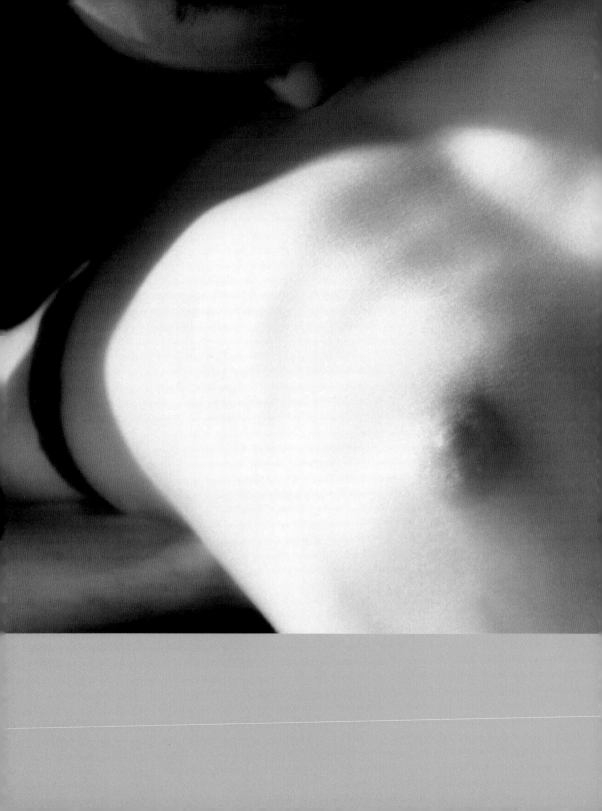

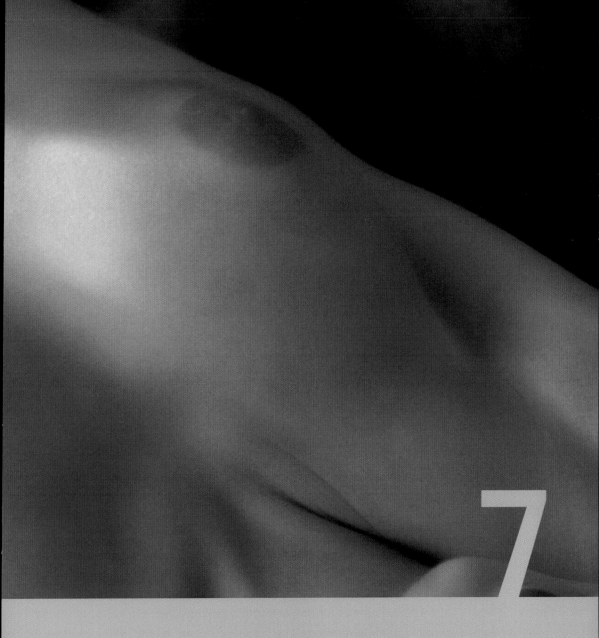

7

A Brave New Sexuality

Considering Change

For the benefit of doubting readers, let's look at why the world won't fall apart should you choose to tolerate the ideas put forward in this book. After all, there must be some risk, mustn't there? If people were allowed to do as they pleased sexually, they might wander naked in the streets and casually fuck in the nearest shop doorway. Surely the world as we know it would fall apart? Wouldn't it? Wouldn't such behaviour mean we had reverted to an animal state? And if we became animal-like again, wouldn't that mean the end of civilized intelligence? It's a doomsday scenario.

But I suspect that sex will turn out to be a bit like fashion. There will always be people who want to be seen as different. These are the ones who will wear the contemporary equivalent of the Emperor's new clothes, and who will make a point of being blatantly sexual. But there will also be some who want to be traditional, who would no more dream of having public sex than they would of going in for body piercing. Thanks to the balance between the extremes and the 'trads', we wouldn't see huge differences. Far from civilization falling apart, it would simply shift a little. We might achieve some public acceptance of outrageous sex style but we might also see more public rejection of it.

That slight shift in public opinion would probably hit us a little like computers have hit the attention span of young people. Instead of going in for sustained tracts of detailed information, today's readers can only take it in short, sharp bites. This doesn't mean that civilisation is on the decline. It means instead that brains are sharpening up. Young men and women can take in a lot of material more rapidly than the preceding generation provided it is served up to them in small bites rather than large tracts. This isn't decline, but it is change. Sexual ideas change, too.

We Are Human Therefore We Change

Change is the only thing which is inevitable. Just by living and breathing we change. Surely it is better to tolerate and understand change rather than block it or attack it because we are frightened? Indeed, whichever side you happen to be on in the evolutionary ideas war, change is the very basis of any version of evolution. We are human therefore we change.

Judging from recent rapid transformations in scientific discovery, our grandchildren and their descendents are due for some very remarkable choices where sexual options are concerned. On the basis of present technological development, presented here, in light-hearted fashion, are some of the sexual enterprises that could well evolve. In the future, you may be able to:

Change your orgasm Sexual libido (sex drive) has only very recently begun to be understood. It's not beyond the realms of fantasy to envisage a future where you might decide if you want your orgasm to be long and dreamy, shallow and drifting, hard and intense, or rapidly explosive. How could you manage this? By taking a pill appropriately calibrated to release or inhibit sexual energy. Your pill pack might be packaged in the colours of the rainbow, with violet and indigo for rapidly explosive climax, and yellow leading into white for shallow and drifting orgasm. The pills themselves would work on your excitement/inhibition brain centres but would also be boosted with graduated amounts of testosterone to provide additional sensitivity.

Change your sex drive If you hate the idea of swallowing pills containing substances that have to pass through your liver, you might opt for one of the new Booster Sex gels designed to be rubbed directly onto the genitals. These gels would deliver sexual arousal directly to the penile or clitoral area, thus massively sensitizing the area and would also pass into the bloodstream travelling up to the sexual brain centres. The end result: someone who turns on with anyone, under any circumstances. Such a gel would be invaluable to the many women who find it hard to experience orgasm. It would also work wonders for aging men who experience less penile sensitivity and who therefore have problems turning on and sustaining an erection.

Reminder. Only 30 per cent of women can climax
from intercourse alone.

Change your physical shape If you have enough money, you can already do this thanks to plastic surgery. In future, however, not only will you retain the option to totally resculpt your body, but new preparatory drugs will prepare the body to react well to the knife so that you can heal without scarring.

Hardly a month goes by at the time of writing this book when some new discovery isn't made with regards to drugs that prevent the human body from rejecting foreign tissue. It is becoming possible to graft all manner of organs onto human beings, which far from being

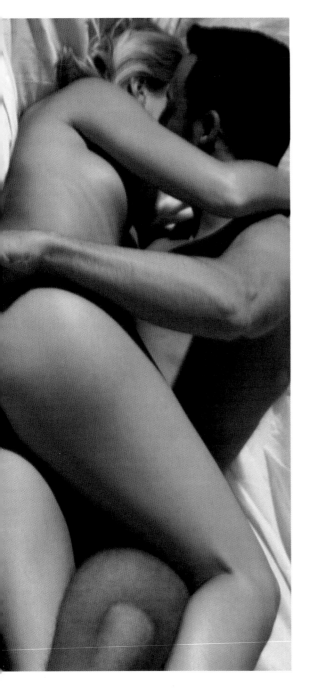

rejected, appear to set like concrete. In future, these spare parts may be grown from our own cloned cell nuclei, so that they would not be rejected as foreign tissue but would instead be welcomed as the body's own.

The sexual possibilities are major. From replacement genitals to somebody else's genitals, to extra genitals over and above the usual set, all of these transplants become logically possible. Imagine a human woman, for example, with sensually enhanced breasts By stroking her new Sensi-Breasts and Sensi-Nipples, she could experience powerful climaxes any time she wanted. Imagine a male with an extra penis, specially designed to penetrate anally, at the same time as his usual penis penetrates vaginally. It's the Sex Aids business gone cosmetic.

Choose the sexuality of your unborn child

And no, I don't mean the gender. I mean the sexuality – the degree to which any child may relate sexually. This would include their libido, their sensitivity, their easy arousal and their expression of sexuality. All it would take would be a small hormonal Sexual Success implant. So that there could be no danger of such a child being perversely exploited, the implant could be timed to come on at an appropriate age. In other words, you could ensure that your child would have no difficulties in enjoying a full sexual life even if you as an adult didn't manage it.

Fuck one person Many of the problems with relationships arise from the fact that one partner (or even both) becomes sexually restless. Perfectly good marriages end because one member of the couple feels virtually compelled to explore the field. Imagine a world where, on marriage, you could choose the option of being bio-emotionally tailored to one other. What would this entail? You could choose to submit yourselves to a method of brain programming so that certain brain pathways regarding sexual attraction in both partners were induced to match perfectly and to focus specifically on each other. This would make it virtually impossible to stray.

The gain would be that many more couples would stay happy together. The loss would show up when one member of the partnership dies. We already see a widow or widower's version of this in the sex therapy clinic, where the bereaved individual wants to be sexual with his/her new partner. This person is indeed strongly attracted to the new lover, but when it comes to sex, remembers the deceased partner so automatically that sex in the present becomes impossible.

Fuck many people simultaneously Cybersex ultimately makes it possible not only to communicate by webcam but also to wire your body into the internet system by virtue of electrodes attached to specific erogenous zones. This enables you and your partner to experience physical arousal even though you are love-making at extreme long distance. One of the many benefits of this is that you can wire up to more than one individual at a time, a kind of Chat Bedroom where you can take part in orgies.

The advantages would be massively increased sexual experience, particularly for certain people who might not otherwise enjoy a sex life. The disadvantage would be hard wiring – you might get so addicted to the Chat Bedroom that you couldn't leave it. Sad cases would be found holed up in their computer rooms, starved to death but having gasped their last with a look of intense pleasure on their face.

Join the Borg. Fuck the world Trekkies will recognize the reference. The Borg is a race of half-humans, half-automatons who are all plugged into a global brain. They are one of the interesting enemies created for humans to battle in the *Star Trek* TV series. They operate as a hive and roam the universe looking for other races to plug into their system so that their own brains expand and other races are enriched by the enormously varied experience that the Borg can provide.

It's not difficult to extrapolate from the kind of cyber-connections we will soon be able to make that there will be a real possibility of not just joining a small group for virtual sex but, ultimately, of joining an absolutely massive group for Solar Sex. Imagine a society where every member experienced their own and each other's orgasms simultaneously!

The advantage. A massive increase of personal knowledge and orgasms so powerful they could knock you out for days. The disadvantage. Loss of personal identity, autonomy and group vulnerability where if one of you suffers so does everyone.

Download your sex Human beings may reach the stage of having a computer implant attached to the brain at a very early age. One by-product of this is that you could download your evening's sex directly from the internet. You have effectively become the Borg.

The world of floating gender Since our identities may be plugged into other people's brains from an early age, we will find it difficult to remain fixed as either masculine or feminine since our actual experience will be of all genders. This means that not only would we have far greater toleration of differing gender groups but that we might become so tolerant we lose sight of our own gender and become free-floating. Put simply, we would be whatever gender was deemed appropriate for a particular sexual assignment.

The Cyber Ice Age Thanks to a cataclysmic event, the internet is destroyed, leaving the human race to flounder. Civilization will be destroyed, millions will die and the human race will have to begin all over again. Only this time, the great apes may hold the advantage over man since they will know how to survive in the wild. Man, on the other hand, will have virtually lost touch with reality.

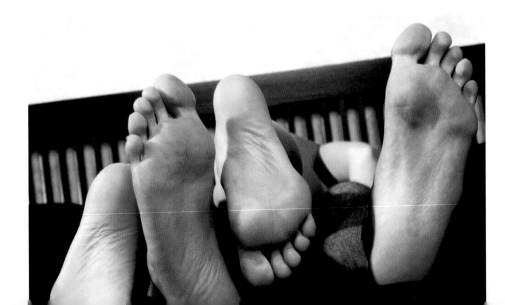

EPILOGUE

At the end of the day, we have choices about how we can experience sex. We don't have to be channelled into what the current belief system puts out. If you go back to evolutionary premises, sex can be anything. It can be old brain (unconscious, instinctive) or it can be new brain (conscious, thoughtful). Either way of experiencing sex is 'real' and 'natural', which is why human beings would be wise to make the most of what they've got. So if sex doesn't feel particularly satisfactory, try rethinking it.

To sum up, rethinking involves:
- Understanding memes – the power of ideas, where they come from, and considering floating a few memes of your own.
- Getting insight into your behaviour and feelings. This means understanding your family background and why you grew up with the personal 'survival' system that affects your sexual choices.
- Deciding if you really want to change or if, in fact, your present situation suits you.
- Making small changes (if that's what you want). Make them gradually but persistently.
- Taking a shot at changing your sexual attitudes. Start off with our mini attitude restructuring section and consider subscribing to one of the bigger ones in San Francisco or starting your own SAR group, where you discuss sexual attitudes so that you get more comfortable with all aspects of sex.
- Making a point of seeing the other side of a sex problem. Take a look at what the problem is trying to tell you about yourself and your relationship.
- Working consciously on feeling happy about what you have got.
- Taking on board the historic perspective – the fact that every generation feels slightly different about sexuality and accordingly behaves differently.
- Deliberately looking at your sex life as if the glass were 'half-full'. Appreciate the creativity that goes into your every sex act and the subtlety of what you have already established with your partner.
- Working on feeling unafraid to pursue the sexual lifestyle that is right for you.

There are no standards for good sex in your brain. Sex is purely what you make it. On the other hand, remembering the story of the Moon orbiting around the Sun, sex is always, well, just...sex.

Bibliography

Bagemihl, Bruce, *Biological Exuberance*, St Martins Press, New York, 1999.

Bancroft, John. *Human Sexuality and its Problems*, Churchill Livingstone, Edinburgh, London, Melbourne and New York, 1989.

Blackmore, Susan, *The Meme Machine*, OUP, Oxford, 2000.

Evans, Dylan and Zarate, Oscar, *Introducing Evolutionary Psychology*, Icon, London and New York, 1999.

Hawes, Clair, *Couples Growing Together, – a marriage enrichment program*, Coast Center for Mediation and Counseling, Vancouver, 1997.

Holford, Jeremy and Hooper, Anne, *Adler for Beginners*, Writers and Readers, London and New York, 1998.

Hooper, Anne, *The Body Electric*, Virago, London, 1979.

Hooper, Anne, *Kama Sutra*, Dorling Kindersley, London and New York, 2000.

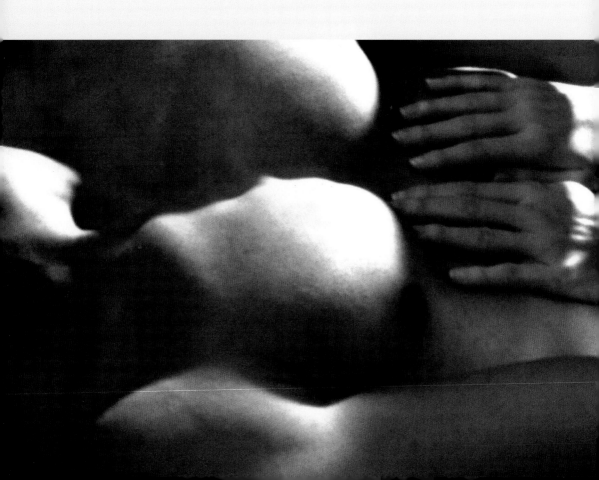

Hooper, Anne and Perring, Michael, *Get Fit, Feel Fantastic*, Carroll & Brown, London, 2000.

Kinsey, Pomeroy, Martin, *Sexual Behaviour in the Human Male*, Saunders, Philadelphia and London, 1948.

Lovell, Mary, *A Rage to Live: A Biography of Richard and Isabel Burton*, Norton, New York, 2000.

Masters, William and Johnson, Virginia, *Homosexuality in Perspective*, Little, Brown and Co, Boston, 1979.

Miller, Geoffrey, *The Mating Mind*, Heineman, London, 2000.

National Sex Forum, *SAR Guide for a Better Sex Life*, National Sex Forum, San Francisco, 1977.

Rose, Hilary and Rose, Steven, *Alas Poor Darwin*, Jonathan Cape, London, 2000.

Stopes, Marie, *Married Love*, Reprinted Phoenix Press, US, 2000.

Storr, Anthony, *The Dynamics of Creation*, Penguin, London, 1972.

Wellings, Kaye et al, *Sexual Behaviour in Britain*, Penguin, London, 1994.

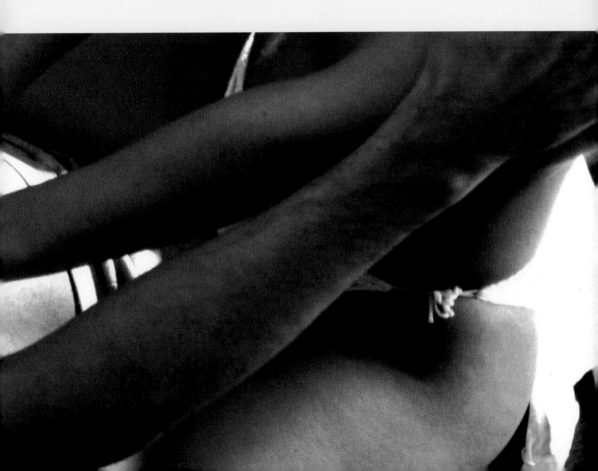

APPENDIX

For more information on Sexual Attitude Restructuring (SAR) courses, write to the Institute for the Advanced Study of Human Sexuality, 1523 Franklin Street, San Francisco, CA 94109 USA Tel: (415) 928-1133

or go to their website: www.iashs.edu

For self-teaching material on how to experience orgasm, look out for *The Body Electric* written by myself (see bibliography, page 158) available by mail order from P.O. Box 29742, London NW3 1FF. Cheque for £10.00 (includes postage and packing) should be made out to Anne Hooper.

ACKNOWLEDGMENTS

*To my colleagues Jeremy Holford-Miettinen
and Dr Michael Perring for the information and stimulation they
have supplied on the subject of sex and evolution.*

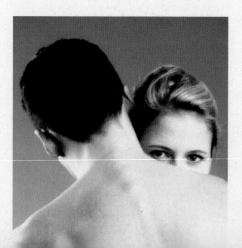